Case Presentations in Anaesthesia and Intensive Care

Kenneth J. Power, BM, MRCP, FCAnaes
Consultant in Anaesthesia and Intensive Care,
Poole General Hospital, Poole, Dorset

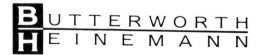

BUTTERWORTH
HEINEMANN

To Jamie, Becky and Charlie

Butterworth-Heinemann Ltd
Linacre House, Jordan Hill, Oxford OX2 8DP

 PART OF REED INTERNATIONAL BOOKS

OXFORD   LONDON   BOSTON
MUNICH   NEW DELHI   SINGAPORE   SYDNEY
TOKYO   TORONTO   WELLINGTON

First published 1992
Reprinted 1992

British Library Cataloguing in Publication Data
A catalogue record for this book is available from the British Library

Library of Congress Cataloguing in Publication Data
A catalogue record for this book is available from the Library of Congress

ISBN 0 7506 0497 2

Printed and bound in Great Britain by
Redwood Press, Melksham, Wiltshire

Preface

Candidates studying for postgraduate medical examinations often find that learning from case histories provides an enjoyable break from some of the drudgery of textbook revision. Despite a plethora of such books relating to medicine and surgery there is a relative dearth of such collections in the fields of anaesthesia and intensive care. The purpose of this volume is to attempt to rectify some of that imbalance.

This book consists of 31 case presentations on topics related to anaesthesia and intensive care. Each consists of a short history and the findings from physical examination, supported where appropriate by electrocardiograms, chest X-rays, laboratory results and other investigations. This is followed by a series of questions arising from the case; these are aimed at highlighting areas that are perhaps difficult (or subject to difficulties in understanding or conception), topical or even controversial. These themes are then developed in the subsequent dicussion. In this way each case acts as a catalyst from which other areas may be developed; a tack often taken by examiners in the clinical and viva sections of the examination.

In such a relatively small book the discussions are not intended to be exhaustive reviews of each and every topic mentioned, but rather aim to address a wide variety of issues, alerting the reader to areas where further thought or reading might prove valuable. The underlying approach is to underpin clinical practice with a clear understanding of the relevant physiology and pharmacology and to provide an appreciation of how these may be modified by disease states and coexisting medical conditions.

The book is not exclusively aimed at candidates for any particular part of the Fellowship examination but will hopefully provide something of interest to anaesthetists at all stages of their clinical training, and maybe also to those from other specialties who have an input to intensive and high care units.

I am indebted to a number of consultants at Southampton General Hospital, notably Paul Spargo, Rick Lawes, Mick Nielsen and David Laycock, who have reviewed cases relating to their particular fields of interest and provided a number of helpful suggestions in terms of refining the text.

Finally, do enjoy the book! Please write with your comments – and good luck with whatever examinations you may happen to be taking.

Kenneth J. Power

Case 1

A 40-year-old woman with long-standing rheumatoid arthritis required bilateral Keller's osteotomies. She had widespread joint involvement and completed a course of steroids 3-months previously following an acute flare-up of her condition. Her current medication consisted of aspirin 1 g three times daily, sodium aurothiomalate 20 mg weekly (total of 60 mg this course) and ferrous sulphate (Feospan) 150 mg daily.

Examination revealed widespread articular involvement, thin skin and easy bruising. No cardiovascular abnormalities were discovered. Investigation of the respiratory tract showed dullness to percussion and reduced air entry at the right lung base. The spleen was palpable. Laboratory investigations showed a haemoglobin level of 8.9 g/dl, a white blood cell count of 1.5×10^9/l and a platelet count of 75×10^9/l. Urea and electrolyte values were sodium 130 mmol/l, potassium 3.7 mmol/l, urea 9.5 mmol/l, bicarbonate 28 mmol/l, and creatinine was 170 µmol/l. Radiographs of the chest and cervical spine are shown in *Figures 1a–c*.

Questions

1. What possible explanations are there for this woman's anaemia? Would you give a transfusion preoperatively?
2. What do the X-rays show? Does the chest X-ray finding warrant any action?
3. What would be your anaesthetic technique and why?
4. What regional technique could you employ to provide postoperative analgesia, and which nerves would need to be blocked? Does the fact that the operation is bilateral pose a problem?
5. Would you favour the use of a non-steroidal anti-inflammatory drug for postoperative analgesia in this patient?

Discussion

Patients with rheumatoid arthritis are generally anaemic and this may result from a number of causes. Firstly there is the normochromic, normocytic anaemia of any chronic disease. Secondly, therapy with salicylates, non-steroidal anti-inflammatory drugs and

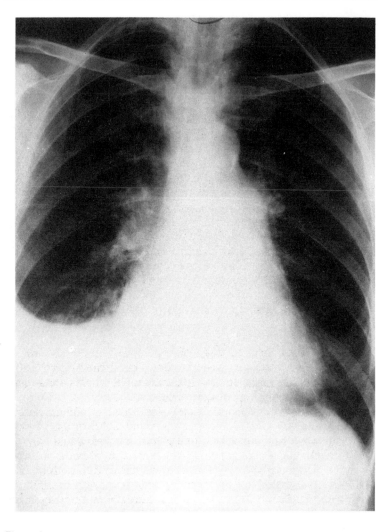

Figure 1a

possibly also steroids will result in gastric erosion or ulceration and the development of iron deficiency anaemia from chronic blood loss. Less commonly, severe rheumatoid disease can lead to amyloid deposition within the kidney resulting in impaired renal function and the anaemia of renal failure (erythropoietin deficien-

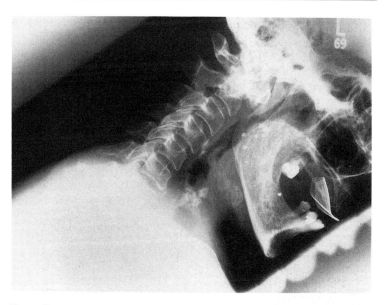

Figure 1b

cy). Renal complications may be compounded by the use of potentially nephrotoxic agents such as non-steroidal anti-inflammatory drugs, gold and penicillamine. In this case gold therapy may have caused a pancytopenia rather than the more common agranulocytosis, but the presence of splenomegaly makes a further cause of anaemia in rheumatoid disease likely: Felty's syndrome. This is the combination of rheumatoid arthritis and splenomegaly with anaemia and thrombocytopenia.

There would be little point in transfusing this patient to a haemoglobin level greater than 10 g/dl; for surgery such as multiple foot osteotomies, performed under tourniquet and with little anticipated blood loss, a good case can be made for accepting this level of haemoglobin.

The cervical spine X-rays (*Figures 1b, 1c*) show what is probably the most worrying concern to the anaesthetist when approaching a patient with rheumatoid arthritis: atlantoaxial subluxation. The odontoid peg, the tip of which is eroded in this case, is attached to the anterior arch of the atlas (C-1) by a transverse ligament. Evidence of subluxation is said to be present when the space between the anterior arch of C-1 and the odontoid is greater

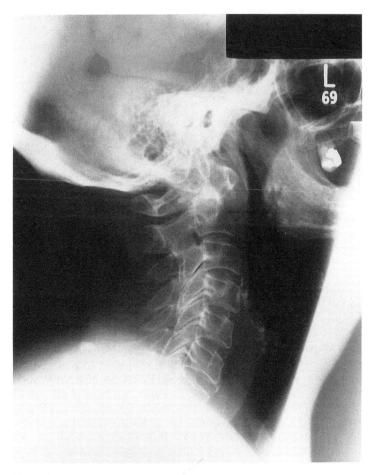

Figure 1c

than 5 mm (3–5 mm is equivocal). Note the increase in the gap when the film is taken in flexion. Remember 'Steel's rule of three' which states that one-third of the arch of the atlas is occupied by the odontoid anteriorly, one-third by the cervical cord posteriorly and one-third by the intervening space. There is thus some room for the odontoid to move posteriorly relative to the atlas (C-1) without jeopardizing the cord; but excess head and neck movement, as might occur at intubation, carries the risk of cord transection.

The chest X-ray (*Figure 1a*) shows a small right pleural effusion which should be left alone as it is not compromising respiratory function. As a rule of thumb, pleural effusions occupying one-third to one-half of a hemithorax probably warrant preoperative drainage.

Spinal anaesthesia would be the method of choice in this patient, although it might be technically difficult to perform. Steroid cover is indicated as she has been taking these drugs in the last 6 months. If general anaesthesia is required intubation should be avoided, and indeed, there is no indication for it. Mask anaesthesia is entirely appropriate; in any case the neck should be supported in a collar; and great care taken with patient transfer, etc. If it was felt that the airway would be particularly difficult to maintain a Brain laryngeal mask could prove useful.

A five-nerve ankle block could provide excellent analgesia in this patient. The five nerves to be blocked are the posterior tibial nerve behind the medial malleolus and posterior to the posterior tibial artery; the saphenous nerve (the sensory continuation of the femoral nerve) in front of the medial malleolus; the sural nerve running behind the lateral malleolus; the deep peroneal nerve (supplying the web between the great and second toe) medial to the dorsalis pedis artery on the dorsum of the foot, and the branches of the superficial peroneal nerve (by injecting a subcutaneous band superficial to the extensor retinaculum along the lateral half of a line joining the two malleoli). It is important to remember to perform the block prior to inflation of the tourniquets to avoid the risk of intravascular injection. Incidentally, when tourniquets are used in patients with fragile skin it is probably best to avoid the shearing stresses produced by Esmarch bandages.

The problem with performing the block bilaterally is that blocking ten nerves requires a considerable amount of local analgesic and care needs to be taken to avoid toxic doses.

Non-steroidal anti-inflammatory drugs (NSAIDs) such as diclofenac exert their analgesic effect through the inhibition of cyclooxygenase. The pain associated with peripheral tissue damage is mediated by bradykinin and other products of arachidonic acid metabolism and potentiated by prostaglandins. Arachidonic acid may be metabolized by one of two pathways: via the cyclooxygenase pathway to prostaglandins, prostacyclin and thromboxane; or via the lipo-oxygenase pathway leading to the production of the leukotrienes (e.g. interleukin VI). These drugs would appear to provide effective surgical analgesia following many minor and intermediate procedures without the attending problems of sedation and respiratory depression associated with the opiates. NSAIDs are generally highly protein bound with reduced clearances in elderly patients. However, the surge in enthusiasm for their use should be tempered with caution, particularly in patients with evidence of renal impairment. Although not solely responsible, prostaglandins are important as mediators of autoregulation in the renal vascular bed particularly under conditions of vasoconstriction and reduced renal blood flow. The drugs appear to be safe provided the patient is well hydrated and not dependent on prostaglandins for renal blood flow autoregulation. However, prostaglandin autoregulation may be particularly important in patients with hypovolaemia, congestive cardiac failure and hepatic cirrhosis, and it would seem prudent to avoid the use of NSAIDs in these circumstances and in patients with preoperative evidence of renal impairment and perhaps those taking diuretics.

There is recent interest in the use of combined analgesic regimens where combinations of opiates, NSAIDs and regional blocks may be used additively and synergistically to optimize analgesia. Pretreatment with NSAIDs prior to surgery may have a role in preventing the stimulation and sensitization of peripheral nociceptors prior to surgical trauma.

Case 2

A 72-year-old man was a known hypertensive and had suffered two previous myocardial infarctions, 3 and 4 years previously. Since then he has experienced intermittent angina of variable severity. At a 6-monthly check his general practitioner noted a pulse of 50 beats/min and changed his antihypertensive medication from atenolol to captopril. A pulsatile abdominal mass was also discovered and the patient was referred to a vascular surgeon. A subsequent ultrasound examination confirmed the presence of a 6-cm abdominal aortic aneurysm. The patient's medication consisted of captopril, 25 mg twice daily; nifedipine 10 mg three times daily; frusemide 40 mg once daily and spironolactone 100 mg once daily, with glyceryl trinitrate spray when required.

On examination the patient was found to have a pulse of 48 beats/min with dropped beats, and blood pressure of 150/85 mmHg. No other physical signs were found. Laboratory investigations showed a haemoglobin level of 16 g/dl, a white cell count of $8.0 \times 10^9/l$ and a platelet count of $320 \times 10^9/l$. Urea and electrolyte values were sodium 132 mmol/l, potassium 5.5 mmol/l, urea 12 mmol/l, bicarbonate 26 mmol/l and creatinine 205 µmol/l. The electrocardiogram is shown in *Figure 2a*.

Questions

1. How does captopril exert its hypotensive action? What explanations can you offer for the moderately elevated values of urea, creatinine and potassium?
2. Discuss whether the patient should be offered elective repair of his aortic aneurysm.
3. What was the cause of his bradycardia? Should any special investigations or procedures be carried out preoperatively?
4. What intraoperative monitoring would you require and at what points in the surgery do you think it would be most valuable?
5. Would the patient's condition and medication influence your choice of volatile agent?

Discussion

Captopril is an angiotensin converting enzyme inhibitor. When low perfusion is detected by the renal juxtaglomerular apparatus the physiological response is the release of renin, which leads to angiotensin I production and the enzymatic formation of angiotensin II in the lung. Angiotensin II is a potent vasoconstrictor, with the effect of elevating the arterial pressure. In the face of a low renal perfusion pressure angiotensin II causes vasoconstriction of the efferent glomerular arteriole, so maintaining the glomerular filtration pressure. By blocking this mechanism captopril may cause an elevation of the urea and creatinine. Spironolactone can cause some deterioration in renal function and the aldosterone antagonist action of spironolactone could account for the hyperkalaemia. Remember that long-standing hypertension per se may result in a deterioration of renal function.

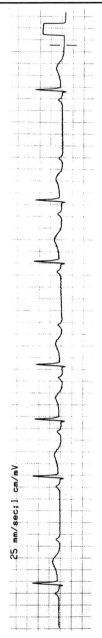

25 mm/sec; 1 cm/mV

Figure 2a

Whether the patient should be offered surgery is essentially a cost–benefit analysis of the advantages that are likely to result set against the risks. The most reliable prognostic indicator for future rupture is aneurysm size. Patients with an aneurysm 6 cm in diameter have a 5-year survival rate of only 6% and half of those deaths will be due to rupture of the aneurysm; it must be borne in mind that the operative mortality rate of emergency aneurysm surgery remains in excess of 50%, whereas the mortality for elective repair is around 2%. Following successful repair of an aneurysm, mortality is no different from other groups matched for age and medical condition. Almost by definition, all patients with abdominal aortic aneurysms are arteriopaths with coronary atheroma, and the majority of deaths in the perioperative period will be from myocardial infarction. One of the most quoted indices of cardiac risk is that described by Goldmann, who allocated point scores to various risk factors (*Tables 2a, 2b*). This patient would

Table 2a   Risk factor scores for calculating the Goldman cardiac risk index

Risk factor	Points
Third heart sound or raised jugular venous pressure	11
Myocardial infarct within 6 months	10
More than 5 ventricular ectopic beats per minute	7
Rhythm other than sinus	7
Age greater than 70 years	5
Intraperitoneal, thoracic or aortic surgery	3
Emergency	4
Aortic stenosis	3
Poor general condition	3

Table 2b   The Goldman cardiac risk index

Class	Points	Nil or minor complications (%)	Life-threatening complications (%)	Cardiac death (%)
I	0–5	99	0.7	0.2
II	6–12	93	5	2
III	13–25	86	11	2
IV	25+	22	22	56

score 18 points and thus falls within class III, with an 86% chance of an uneventful course and a 2% mortality. It would therefore seem appropriate to offer him surgery.

The ECG shows second-degree heart block of the Mobitz I variety (Wenckebach phenomenon) where a progressive lengthening of the PR interval eventually leads to a dropped beat. This is generally considered a relatively benign condition but could progress to complete heart block under surgery and anaesthesia. The patient should probably have a temporary cardiac pacemaker inserted beforehand. Another possibility would be to use a Swan-Ganz catheter with a pacing channel to permit pacing of the right ventricle if required.

Many centres would accept such a patient for repair without further special investigations. However, others might argue that the state of the coronary arteries should be assessed beforehand with coronary angiography and, if necessary, a coronary artery bypass graft performed prior to aortic surgery. It has been suggested that if appropriate patients receive coronary grafts prior to aortic surgery then the overall mortality may be half that if abdominal aneurysm surgery alone had been undertaken.

The ejection fraction could be measured and ventricular wall motion assessed non-invasively using a radionucleotide ventriculogram. An ejection fraction of less than 40% should lead to serious questions about the wisdom of operating.

In a cardiovascularly fit patient a central venous pressure line is probably adequate monitoring. However, in a patient with impaired cardiovascular function and a relatively non-compliant vascular tree, due to long-standing hypertension, there is likely to be poor and unpredictable toleration of the stresses of induction, aortic cross-clamping and unclamping. In this situation a Swan-Ganz catheter with the facility to measure cardiac output and systemic vascular resistance will offer the ability to control the filling pressure of the left ventricle with appropriate volume replacement and permit precise and logical manipulation of the circulation with inotropes, vasoconstrictors and vasodilators as appropriate.

Aortic cross-clamping may increase the systemic vascular resistance by up to 30%. The diseased, ischaemic myocardium may be unable to cope with this increase in 'afterload' and cardiac output may fall. As the heart fails, the left ventricular end-diastolic pressure (LVEDP) — reflected by the pulmonary artery occlusion pressure (PAOP or 'wedge') — will tend to rise, reducing the coronary perfusion pressure (LVEDP minus diastolic pressure). A vicious circle of falling cardiac output and myocardial ischaemia will then develop. This could be countered by an intravenous vasodilator such as glyceryl trinitrate to reduce the resistance against which the left ventricle is ejecting, dilate the coronary arteries and restore a more favourable balance between myocardial oxygen supply and demand. When the cross-clamp is ready to be released, vasodilators should be discontinued and rapid volume infusion anticipated to counter the increase in the intravascular space with unclamping.

Attenuating the renal damage that may occur during the cross-clamp period is important, particularly where preoperative renal function is suboptimal; renal dopamine at around 3 µg/kg per minute has been shown to be beneficial.

Thoracic epidural blockade is frequently used in these patients to provide postoperative analgesia. The use of bupivacaine to block the sympathetic outflow of the thoracic dermatomes will produce vasodilatation, but the extent of the block may be unpredictable and the hypotension harder to reverse than when provided by specific vasodilators. However, epidural blockade can provide a 'stress-free' operative field and effective postoperative analgesia, which may have beneficial effects on the balance of myocardial oxygen supply and demand in the postoperative period.

Isoflurane is arguably contraindicated in patients with ischaemic heart disease who are also receiving nifedipine. Isoflurane is a potent coronary vasodilator and as such is suspected of causing a coronary steal phenomenon where the dilatation of normal coronary vessels diverts blood away from diseased or maximally dilated vessels, rendering their territory of supply even more ischaemic. The case is, however, not conclusively proven, and against this must be set the benefits of isoflurane in that it is less negatively inotropic than the other volatile agents.

Nifedipine exerts its vasodilatory effect through calcium channel blockade and it is believed that the vasodilatory effects of isoflurane are exerted through similar mechanisms. It can be argued that the use of the two agents together may result in excessive vasodilatation and hypotension.

Case 3

The patient in case 2 underwent an uneventful operative course. He was extubated at the end of the procedure and was transferred to a high-care area breathing 40% oxygen via a face mask. Postoperative analgesia was to be provided by means of a thoracic epidural block delivering an opiate. After 48 hours, however, this patient had produced less than 500 ml of urine in total.

The patient was observed to have a regular pulse of 70 beats/mins, and his blood pressure was 150/90 mmHg. The central venous pressure was 15 mmHg; this increased to 18 mmHg after 250 ml of albumin solution was administered, but there was no change in the urine output. Laboratory investigations showed the following values:

Serum sodium 130 mmol/l, potassium 5.0 mmol/l, chloride 100 mmol/l, bicarbonate 24/mmol/l
Urea 23 mmol/l
Creatinine 300 μmol/l
Plasma osmolality 302 mosmol/kg
Urine osmolality 310 mosmol/kg
Urinary electrolytes: sodium 80 mmol/l, potassium 10 mmol/l

Questions

1. For how long would you continue postoperative oxygen therapy in this man?
2. What would your choice of opiate be in this man? What are the hazards of epidural opiates? What are the ideal properties of an opiate for epidural administration?
3. What is the nature of this man's oliguria? How might it be managed on a general intensive care unit?

Discussion

It is becoming increasingly recognized that episodic hypoxaemia, particularly during sleep, may occur for several days following major surgery and anaesthesia. This may be particularly hazardous in patients with ischaemic heart disease and may well have an important role in the aetiology of myocardial infarction occurring in the first few days postoperatively. A strong case can be made for continuing oxygen therapy for 3 days or so into the postoperative period. The counsel of excellence would be to monitor the arterial oxygen saturation by means of a pulse oximeter.

Side-effects of epidurally administered opiates include nausea and vomiting, urinary retention and pruritus, but by far the most important complication is respiratory depression which may be delayed in onset for over 12 hours following a single bolus injection of epidural morphine. This is brought about by rostral spread of the opiate via the cerebrospinal fluid (CSF) to brain-stem respiratory centres. The chief site of analgesic action for opiates administered epidurally is on opiate receptors found in the substantia gelatinosa of the posterior horn of the spinal cord. To obtain access to these receptors the opiate has to diffuse across the dural membrane into the CSF and then be taken up by the lipophilic cord from the aqueous CSF. Thus a lipid-soluble drug such as fentanyl would be preferable to a water-soluble agent such as morphine, because uptake by the cord from the CSF would be more rapid and more complete. Less opiate would be trapped in the CSF, reducing the risk of a significant amount being carried cephalad to the brain stem.

Patients with pre-existing renal disease are at particular risk of developing renal problems following aortic reconstructive surgery. When faced with an oliguric patient it must be decided whether the patient is hypovolaemic and exhibiting an entirely appropriate response, is merely demonstrating an appropriate, but perhaps somewhat exaggerated, postoperative stress (ADH) response, or is truly developing established renal failure with poor glomerular filtration and loss of tubular ability to elaborate or concentrate the urine. The key to the problem lies in clinical assessment, coupled with simple biochemistry of the plasma *and the urine.* The central venous pressure readings and their response to the fluid challenge with albumin indicate that the problem is not hypovolaemia; further injudicious use of fluids would risk the development of pulmonary oedema which would probably be unresponsive to diuretic therapy owing to the impaired renal function.

The serum urea level has risen by 11 mmol/l and the creatinine level by 95 μmol/l in 48 hours. The urine osmolality indicates a loss of ability to concentrate the urine and a failure to retain sodium (hypovolaemia and postoperative stress are characterized by sodium retention). Potassium excretion is impaired and dangerous hyperkalaemia may develop if the renal failure progresses. The patient therefore is in established acute renal failure and will require some form of renal replacement therapy to:

1. remove fluid, prevent the development of pulmonary and peripheral oedema and allow the administration of essential fluids and nutrients whether enterally or parenterally;
2. remove solutes, fixed acids and other products of metabolism and maintain these at safe levels, and as far as possible preserve the 'milieu intérieur'.

This can be achieved in the general intensive care unit using continuous haemofiltration or possibly haemodiafiltration (*Figure 3a*). This may be accomplished, in principle, by passing the patient's blood through a haemofilter with a pore size that will permit the passage of molecules with a molecular weight up to 30 000. This will result in an ultrafiltrate of plasma containing solutes and electrolytes in the same concentrations that are present in the plasma, and thus the creatinine or urea clearance rate will be equivalent to the filtration rate, typically around 10–15 ml/min. The filtration rate will be proportional to the driving pressure and the vertical distance between the filter and the

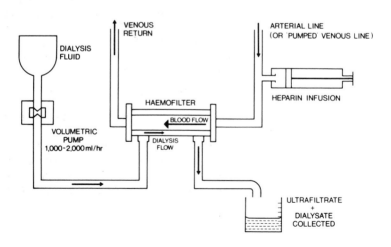

Figure 3a Haemofiltration

collecting vessel, and inversely proportional to the plasma oncotic pressure. In its simplest form the patient's own arterial pressure (if adequate) can be used to pump blood through the filter using cannulae in the femoral artery and vein or a surgically implanted arterio-venous shunt. Femoral lines might be felt to be contraindicated following aortic reconstructive surgery and a veno-veno system using a double lumen subclavian catheter might be preferable; this would require the incorporation of a pump to drive the circuit. The appropriate fluid balance with respect to the volume filtered and other losses is achieved with the use of a haemofiltration replacement fluid. A routine solution would typically be isotonic with similar electrolyte concentrations to plasma, bicarbonate given in the form of acetate or lactate (which require adequate muscle and liver metabolism for their conversion). Filtration rates may be increased by returning the replacement fluid proximal to the filter thus lowering the oncotic pressure of the blood presented to the filter — the so-called technique of pre-dilution.

In a non-catabolic, non-septic patient, filtration alone may achieve adequate homeostasis. However, if required, further solute clearance may be achieved by passing a dialysis solution around the outside of the filter in a direction opposite to the blood flow (countercurrent principle). In this way solutes passing through the filter can diffuse down their concentration gradients into the dialysis fluid which is collected with the filtration fluid. The net removal of fluid will then be the volume collected minus the volume of dialysate given. Solute clearance is now due to a combination of dialysis and filtration. Recent reviews have recommended dialysis flow rates of 1600 ml/h and this should result in creatine clearances of the order of 20–30 ml/h.

Anticoagulation is required and this is generally achieved with a continuous heparin infusion, the rate of which is adjusted in the light of frequent activated clotting times or activated partial thromboplastin ratios.

Prostacyclin is sometimes used as an expensive alternative to heparin, generally if it is felt desirable to exploit the vasodilator properties of this drug or if a significant bleeding problem exists. Prostacyclin is a potent inhibitor of platelet activation and will tend to maintain the platelet count and function.

Case 4

An 18-month-old girl had been unwell with symptoms of an upper respiratory tract infection for 3 days. She was brought to hospital with increasing respiratory difficulty.

On examination the child was found to be febrile (38°C), peripherally cool and pale, with slight central cyanosis. A regular tachycardia of 160 beats/min was observed, together with loud inspiratory stridor, tracheal tug, intercostal recession and indrawing. The child was drooling at the mouth and had a barking cough. A full blood count revealed levels of haemoglobin 13 g/dl, white cells 18×10^9/l and platelets 240×10^9/l. The chest radiograph is shown in *Figure 4a*. Arterial blood gas measurement was attempted but failed.

Questions

1. Comment on the investigations; do you think they were appropriate?
2. What is the differential diagnosis and which is most likely in this child?
3. Describe precisely how you would overcome the problem.
4. How would you subsequently manage the child; spontaneous respiration or ventilation? What type of circuit or ventilator? What monitoring would you institute and does it have any limitations?
5. Comment on the position of the tubes inserted into the child.
6. How would you manage the extubation?

Discussion

None of the investigations performed influences the immediate management of this child who clinically has symptoms and signs of severe upper airways obstruction requiring rapid relief. Venepuncture and repeated attempts at obtaining blood gases will result in distress and crying, increasing oxygen requirements to a level which it may not be possible to meet in the presence of severe airflow obstruction.

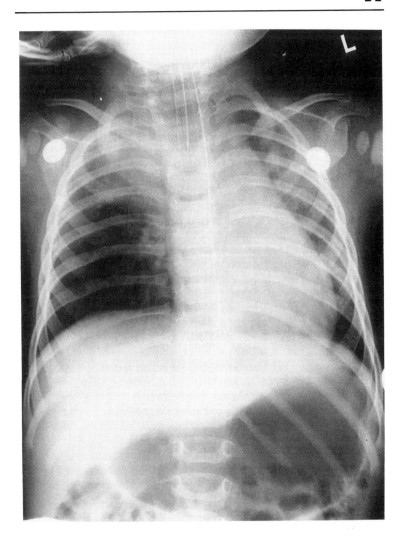

Figure 4a

The diagnosis lies between acute laryngotracheal bronchitis (croup) and acute epiglottitis. Croup is the more likely diagnosis here. Epiglottitis tends to occur in older children (3–8 years), but can occur at any age. The onset of symptoms is generally very acute, over hours rather than days, and the child is markedly unwell, toxic and febrile. In this child there is upper lobe collapse and consolidation on the chest X-ray which is much more likely to occur with croup; in acute epiglottitis the underlying lungs are generally normal. Acute epiglottitis is due to bacterial infection, usually *Haemophilus*; croup is a viral process usually due to parainfluenza or respiratory syncytial viruses.

As stressed before, if the clinical impression is such that the degree of airway obstruction is regarded as critical then the immediate necessity is to intubate the trachea. A clear approach to how this should be done is important. Perhaps most vital is the need not to distress the child. Allow the child to sit up on the mother's knee while introducing halothane in 100% oxygen; only tightly applying the face mask when the child is asleep. As anaesthesia deepens, oxygen consumption falls and arterial saturations should improve. Patience is needed to ensure the child is deeply anaesthetized prior to any attempts at instrumentation of the airway. It is important to appreciate that it may take up to half an hour to achieve an adequate depth of anaesthesia and then a good rule of thumb is to continue 5% halothane for a further 5 minutes. Venous access should be deferred until this stage, at which point atropine 20 μg/kg would be appropriate. When anaesthesia is sufficiently deep, intubation should be performed, with a range of endotracheal tubes to hand. Neuromuscular blocking agents are strictly contraindicated. An otolaryngologist should be immediately available to perform an emergency tracheostomy. Initial intubation is performed expeditiously via the oral route. Having secured the airway a decision can be made to change this to a nasal tube which is generally easier to secure safely. A nasogastric tube is also passed to decompress the stomach and to permit rehydration and the administration of sedatives via the enteral route. Note in this case the high position of the nasogastric tube and the unrelieved gastric dilatation which would necessitate further advancement of the tube. The endotracheal tube is, however, satisfactorily positioned above the carina.

Subsequent management on the intensive care unit poses a number of problems. Generally, the underlying lungs are relatively normal and do not require mechanical ventilation per se, and spontaneous respiration is preferable in the event of accidental extubation. However, the work of breathing through a small endotracheal tube may be considerable. Added to this is the fact that once the child has recovered from the initial exhaustion, because she is otherwise well and vigorous, large doses of sedative agents may be required to achieve adequate sedation.

Triclofos (50–100 mg/kg) via the nasogastric tube is traditionally used, but may have to be supplemented with intravenous benzodiazepines or opiates. Children of this age should not be allowed to breathe spontaneously through an endotracheal tube open to atmospheric pressure and 5 cm of continuous positive airway pressure should be applied to prevent airway collapse and maintain the functional residual capacity. It may be useful to augment this with one or two mandatory machine breaths each minute. Continuous flow infant ventilators of the T-piece occluder type such as the Babylog and the Sechrist are very useful in this respect.

An arterial line is useful to monitor Pa_{O_2} and Pa_{CO_2}, but persistent attempts in difficult cases are probably unwise. Certainly with regard to oxygenation all the required information can be gained from pulse oximetry if the Fi_{O_2} is low.

End-tidal CO_2 monitoring is more problematic in young children where the end-tidal readings obtained from the capnometer will be subject to considerable dilution due to the high continuous flows used in paediatric circuits.

Extubation should be performed in the same controlled setting as the intubation (preferably in a theatre anaesthetic room). The airway is assessed with the deeply anaesthetized child breathing spontaneously. In epiglottitis, the epiglottis is inspected visually. When the obstruction is subglottic, a useful guide to the timing of extubation is the presence of an audible leak around the tube when subjected to an airway pressure of 20 cmH_2O (assuming an appropriate-sized tube is in situ).

Case 5

A fit and healthy 22-year-old man was admitted to the day care surgical unit for the extraction of two wisdom teeth. He was known to be epileptic but had suffered no fits for 3 years and was not taking any medication. He received no premedication and his anaesthesia was induced intravenously using propofol. Suxamethonium was used to facilitate intubation of the trachea. Anaesthesia was uneventful spontaneously breathing a mixture of nitrous oxide, oxygen and enflurane. While in the recovery area the patient noted some diminution in his hearing, but 2 hours later he appeared to have made a full recovery and was discharged home.

The following day he visited his general practitioner complaining of severe pains in the chest.

Questions

1. Why is propofol preferable to an induction agent such as thiopentone in the day case setting?
2. Comment on the choice of volatile agent.
3. Can you offer an explanation for the sensation of deafness on recovery?
4. What should be ensured prior to discharging the patient and what instructions should be issued?
5. Can you explain the symptoms with which he presents to the general practitioner?
6. How might the chest pains have been avoided?

Discussion

Thiopentone is not an ideal drug for use in the day case setting as its use may be followed by prolonged hangover; this is because the action of the drug is terminated by redistribution rather than metabolism. Being highly lipid-soluble, thiopentone is extensively distributed to the fat, from where it slowly leaches back into the circulation prior to metabolism. Thus subanaesthetic concentrations persist in the blood for a prolonged period after a bolus dose.

By contrast, the action of propofol is largely terminated by metabolism, which in part explains the clear-headed quality of recovery that has come to be associated with its use. Propofol has a biphasic elimination phase with a terminal elimination half-life of 405 minutes. It undergoes conjugation in the liver to an inactive metabolite which is subsequently excreted in the urine; 8 hours after a single dose, only 5% will remain detectable in the non-conjugated form. The clearance of the drug is around 1.5–2 l/min. As this figure is in excess of the normal liver blood flow, this implies that there is an extrahepatic site of metabolism — probably the lung.

Enflurane should probably not have been administered to this patient as, unlike the other volatile agents, it has central stimulant properties and causes an increase in electroencephalographic activity. This is exacerbated by hypocapnia, and the manufacturers recommend that enflurane should not be given to patients with an epileptic predisposition. Isoflurane, although an isomer of enflurane, does not possess this undesirable feature and would be an ideal choice as its low blood/gas solubility of 1.4 will contribute towards a rapid return of consciousness in the day case setting.

The complaint of deafness during recovery could well relate to the diffusion of nitrous oxide into the middle ear cavity. Nitrous oxide is more soluble than nitrogen and there will be a greater influx of nitrous oxide into any air-filled space compared with the corresponding efflux of nitrogen. As a consequence pressure will build up, which can result in distortion of the sound transmission and amplification functions of the three bony ossicles of the middle ear. The same considerations relate to the increase in tracheal cuff pressures and the risk of expanding pneumothoraces when nitrous oxide is employed.

Economic considerations and the advent of newer anaesthetic agents producing more rapid and better quality of recovery has led to a considerable expansion in the scope of surgical work that can be dealt with on a day-case basis. However, if day care is to retain a reputation for high patient acceptability, certain prerequisites should be met prior to patient discharge.

Although a patient may appear to be fully recovered an hour or two following a short anaesthetic, more subtle tests of psychomotor function will reveal considerable cognitive impairment. Bearing this in mind, patients should be warned not to drive until the next day and not to operate potentially dangerous machinery, climb ladders, etc. They should ideally be accompanied home and have someone to care for them for the rest of the day. This is particularly important for the elderly patient; it is frequently social factors that preclude day care rather than medical ones, because age per se is no bar to day surgery.

The patient should be aware of what to expect in terms of pain or discomfort and efforts made to minimize these. Dental surgery often results in discomfort for several days afterwards. This should be explained and the patient encouraged to use the supply of analgesics given prior to discharge. Non-steroidal anti-inflammatory drugs such as diclofenac given early in the course of the procedure are useful in providing analgesia when the patient awakens. Patients should be aware that they can contact their general practitioner in the event of problems and be reassured that if necessary readmission to hospital is always available. These considerations, as much as the purely medical ones, are important if day surgery is to retain a high level of patient acceptability, and perhaps suggest that day care is best carried out in a purpose-built facility.

Chest pains occurring in a young man the day after this anaesthetic are almost certainly due to suxamethonium myalgia, about which he should ideally have been warned. These pains generally involve the large muscle groups of the chest, back and neck. They are most frequent in young patients who are ambulant early. There is a vast literature on a plethora of techniques purporting to reduce or eliminate suxamethonium myalgia. These include small precurarization doses of non-depolarizing muscle relaxants, benzodiazepines, lignocaine, large doses of thiopentone and aspirin. However, the range and diversity of the approaches is not reflected in reliable efficacy, and the only way to avoid this troublesome side-effect is to avoid the drug and restrict its use to those situations where it is strictly indicated.

Case 6

A 23-year-old primigravida noted increased dyspnoea with exertion from 16 weeks of pregnancy. At 26 weeks' gestation she complained of hoarseness of voice and was seen by an otolaryngologist, who diagnosed a left recurrent laryngeal nerve palsy. He referred her to a cardiologist who saw her at 28 weeks' gestation, by which time she was breathless at rest.

The cardiologist noted at his examination a regular pulse of 110 beats/min; blood pressure of 110/70 mmHg; jugular venous pressure elevated 5 cm with a marked parasternal heave; first and second heart sounds with a loud pulmonary component to the second heart sound and a long, early diastolic murmur best heard over the left sternal edge. The ECG is shown in *Figure 6a* and the chest radiograph in *Figure 6b*.

The cardiologist made a diagnosis, instituted anticoagulation with heparin and placed the woman on continuous oxygen therapy for the remainder of the pregnancy. Spontaneous labour occurred at 38 weeks' gestation and heparin was discontinued.

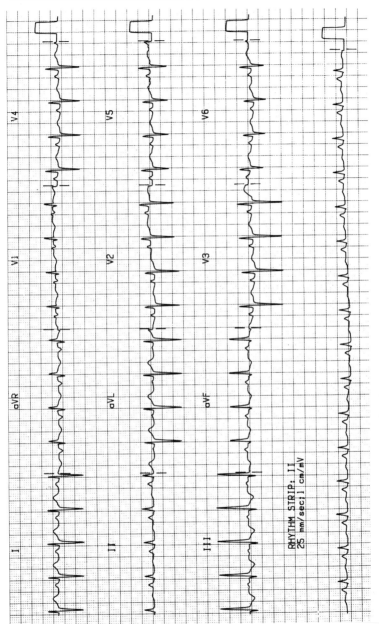

Figure 6a

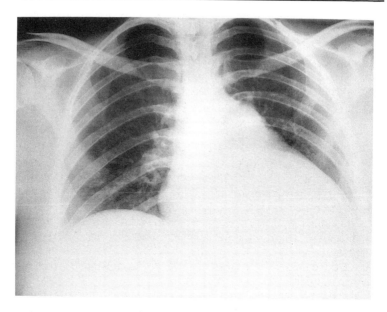

Figure 6b

Questions

1. What is the diagnosis that the cardiologist would have made?
2. Explain the recurrent laryngeal nerve palsy.
3. What would be the best method of providing this patient with analgesia during labour? Discuss the pros and cons and any further monitoring that you might require.
4. General anaesthesia would be very hazardous; if unavoidable, which agents do you think might be preferable?

Discussion

The cardiologist would have made a clinical diagnosis of pulmonary hypertension. The parasternal heave and the loud pulmonary component of the second heart sound are suggestive of right ventricular hypertrophy. The murmur heard is that of tricuspid regurgitation which accounts for the prominent 'v' waves seen in the jugular venous pulse. This is, however, a functional murmur consequent upon the abnormally high pressures in the right side of the heart. The ECG is compatible with the diagnosis with the axis round to the right, evidence of right atrial hypertrophy and poor R wave progression across the anterior chest leads. The chest X-ray shows cardiomegaly with enlargement of the pulmonary conus but with a paucity of vascular markings in the periphery.

The presentation with a right recurrent laryngeal nerve palsy is due to pressure on this nerve as it loops round the enlarged pulmonary hilum.

The definitive diagnosis between primary pulmonary hypertension and secondary pulmonary hypertension due to recurrent pulmonary emboli is notoriously difficult. It is not clear whether pregnancy itself predisposes to the development of pulmonary hypertension or whether the increased demands placed on the cardiovascular system in pregnancy merely unmask a pre-existing condition. Nevertheless, primary pulmonary hypertension in pregnancy has a mortality rate in excess of 50% when the increased cardiac demands of pregnancy are superimposed on what is in effect a fixed cardiac output.

Circulatory collapse may result from a reduction in venous return or a reduction in the systemic vascular resistance, both of which may result from uncontrolled vasodilatation; because of these considerations, spinal or epidural blockade has been traditionally avoided. However, the alternatives — nitrous oxide and opiates — are not effective analgesics in labour, and pain itself is likely to result in dangerous rises in pulmonary vascular resistance due to catecholamine release. Furthermore, nitrous oxide will elevate the pulmonary vascular resistance, as will excessive doses of opiates if these result in hypercapnia. Thus an argument can be made for providing good analgesia by means of a well-controlled epidural block. This will attenuate the increased cardiac demands consequent upon the pain of labour, while also providing the facility for some controlled vasodilatation to accommodate the increased venous return due to placental autotransfusion, which is maximal immediately post partum, when the increase in cardiac output is maximal.

A pulmonary artery catheter would provide valuable information about pulmonary artery pressures; in the event of instability, it would also permit measurement of the pulmonary capillary wedge pressure, the cardiac output and the systemic vascular resistance. However, balloon inflation is particularly hazardous in this group of patients, and the facility should probably only be used if instability develops.

A continuous epidural infusion would be greatly preferable in this setting, avoiding the risk of circulatory collapse with intermittent bolus administration of local anaesthetic agents. Combining an opiate such as fentanyl with bupivacaine could potentiate the analgesic effect and exert a local analgesic sparing effect.

A general anaesthetic would be a very hazardous undertaking. Adequate analgesia for labour could be achieved by obtaining a block to T-10. However, to provide adequate operating conditions for a Caesarean section a block up to T-4, would be required, with a much greater risk of haemodynamic collapse.

As in all pregnant patients undergoing general anaesthesia, a rapid sequence induction would be mandatory. Both the cardio-depressant effects of the induction agents and the catecholamine response to laryngoscopy and intubation are likely to trigger cardiovascular collapse. Isoflurane has been shown to reduce pulmonary vascular resistance in pulmonary hypertensives and may well be the volatile agent of choice, delivered in an air/oxygen mixture to avoid the pressor effect of nitrous oxide on the pulmonary vasculature.

Case 7

A 28-year-old primigravida complained of increasingly painful paraesthesia of the thumb and of the first and second fingers of the left hand. The problem was only noted in the latter weeks of her pregnancy. She was at 32 weeks' gestation and had been previously fit and well.

Examination showed a regular pulse of 95 beats/min; blood pressure 110/70 mm/Hg; first and second heart sounds plus a soft systolic flow murmur best heard in the aortic area. There was slight oedema of the legs. The chest was clear clinically. Laboratory investigations gave the following values:

Haemoglobin 9.9 g/dl
Serum sodium 130 mmol/l, potassium 4.2 mmol/l, chloride 101 mmol/l, bicarbonate 22 mmol/l, urea 2.1 mmol/l
Albumin 29 g/l
Alkaline phosphatase 3 × reference value

24-hour urinary protein excretion 150 mg
Prothrombin time 12 s

Questions

1. Explain the presenting complaint in anatomical terms. What is the root value of the nerve involved and its motor supply in the hand?
2. Is the murmur likely to be of significance?
3. Comment on the normality or otherwise of the investigations.
4. If surgery is deemed necessary, what would you regard as the method of choice for anaesthesia?
5. What factors determine the propensity for a drug such as bupivacaine to accumulate in the fetus?
6. If general anaesthesia was insisted upon, how would you modify your technique compared with the same procedure in a non-pregnant subject?

Discussion

This woman has developed carpal tunnel syndrome, a well-recognized complication of pregnancy. This involves entrapment of the median nerve as it passes under the flexor retinaculum in the wrist. The median nerve is sensory to the thumb, index and middle fingers and the lateral border of the ring finger (the ulnar nerve subserving the rest). It is motor to all the muscles of the thenar eminence with the exception of the adductor pollicis (ulnar), but the only intrinsic hand muscles that it supplies are the lateral two lumbrical muscles.

The systolic murmur is unlikely to be of pathological significance. In normal pregnancy the cardiac output has increased by 40% by the end of the first trimester and continues to rise until term. The increased flow leads to turbulence, and systolic flow murmurs are a common feature of normal pregnancy. Similarly, the presence of oedema has no cardiac connotations and is a feature of normal pregnancy. In isolation oedema does not suggest pre-eclampsia, as this patient is not hypertensive and does not exhibit pathological proteinuria.

The multitude of physiological changes associated with normal pregnancy lead to alterations in the 'normal' ranges for many physiological and biochemical measurements. A haemoglobin level of 10 g/dl is entirely appropriate. Both red cell volume and plasma volume increase during pregnancy, the latter more than the former resulting in a dilutional anaemia. Although there are increased oxygen demands in pregnancy these are more than compensated for by the increase in cardiac output, and the arterial to mixed venous oxygen difference tends to fall.

Normal pregnancy is associated with salt and water retention, a reduced ability to excrete a free water load and a 6-litre expansion of the extracellular fluid. This results in a dilutional hyponatraemia with the serum sodium some 2–3 mmol/l lower than usual, associated with a fall in the plasma osmolality of some 10 mosmol/kg. This, coupled with the increased glomerular filtration rate, lowers the serum urea concentration. The serum albumin drops and there is consequently a fall in the colloid oncotic pressure. This fact, coupled with the increased cardiac demands of pregnancy, renders the pregnant patient particularly at risk of pulmonary oedema formation.

The alkaline phosphatase is normally increased three to fourfold in pregnancy due to placental production.

Because of the risk of the acid aspiration syndrome associated with general anaesthesia in pregnancy, a brachial plexus block would probably be the most suitable anaesthetic technique; and the axillary approach probably is best for hand surgery with the lowest complication rate. Bupivacaine is frequently employed in obstetric practice because of its low fetomaternal ratio (0.3); being long-acting, it will also provide some initial postoperative analgesia. There is a hormonally mediated membrane permeability effect in pregnancy which will tend to increase the likelihood of central nervous system toxicity from amide local anaesthetic agents. Note the somnolence that often occurs in mothers given doses bordering on the upper accepted limit (2 mg/kg) of bupivacaine for epidural Caesarean section.

The propensity for any drug to accumulate in the fetus is dependent upon pH partitioning (ion trapping phenomenon) and the relative protein binding of the drug between the maternal and fetal circulations. Factors such as the placental blood flow and the surface area available for exchange will determine the rate at which the final equilibrium is obtained. Bupivacaine is a base with a pK_a of 8.2, i.e. at a pH of 8.2 half of the drug has accepted a hydrogen ion and become ionized while the other half is in a lipid-soluble free base form and thus able to cross biological membranes. In a more acidic environment a greater proportion will be ionized and unable to cross membranes. Thus when the lipid-soluble base crosses from the mother into the fetus, where the pH is lower (normally around 7.3), a greater proportion is ionized and thus trapped on the fetal side of the circulation. Therefore one would expect bupivacaine to accumulate in the fetus resulting in a fetomaternal ratio greater than one. However, this effect is more than offset by protein binding considerations. Bupivacaine is highly bound to α_1-glycoprotein, levels of which are elevated in the mother but very low in the fetus, in contrast to albumin which is at a higher concentration in the fetus than in the mother. Thus bupivacaine is largely retained in the mother due to protein binding, whereas drugs such as diazepam, extensively bound to the serum albumin, will tend to accumulate in the fetus.

If a general anaesthetic is insisted upon it must be remembered that the patient is at risk of regurgitation and subsequent aspiration of gastric contents, and the usual mask and airway technique employed in a non-pregnant individual would be contraindicated. One in three pregnant women will have evidence of gastric reflux or hiatus hernia at some stage of their pregnancy. It is debatable from what stage of pregnancy a rapid sequence induction becomes obligatory, but 16 weeks would probably be a reasonable answer. Methods should be taken to raise the gastric pH above 2.5 prior to anaesthesia using an H_2-receptor antagonist such as ranitidine, possibly combined with sodium citrate. Due to its evanescent action citrate should be administered no earlier than 20 minutes prior to the induction of anaesthesia. Pregnant patients normally hyperventilate down to a P_{CO_2} of around 30–32 mmHg. The teleological significance of this is the provision of a greater diffusion gradient down which the fetus can eliminate carbon dioxide. Thus spontaneous breathing of anaesthetic agents should only be permitted for the shortest periods; if the surgeon is likely to take 30 minutes or longer the patient should be mechanically ventilated with the aid of a short-acting, non-depolarizing muscle relaxant.

A question mark has been raised over the possible teratogenic effects of nitrous oxide; although a case could be made for avoiding it in the first trimester of pregnancy during the period of organogenesis, this is by no means proven, and is certainly no longer an issue at 32 weeks of gestation.

Case 8

A 25-year-old man was admitted to the accident and emergency department. He had been sitting working under a jacked-up tractor which collapsed on top of him.

On examination the man was found to be agitated, in pain and distress. He was cyanosed but not overtly shocked. There was a regular pulse of 100 beats/min and his blood pressure was 160/100 mmHg. First and second heart sounds were readily heard. Flail segment left chest, reduced air entry left side and coarse crepitations over the right lung field were noted on examination of the chest. Nervous system investigations showed no leg movement to command, flaccid tone and a sensory level demonstrable at D-12.

Questions

1. What are the initial priorities in the resuscitation room?
2. Following insertion of the chest drain, subcutaneous emphysema develops rapidly and vigorous bubbling of the chest drain persists. What diagnosis should be suspected and what procedure is necessary to exclude it? How would you manage the anaesthetic?
3. Would you use suxamethonium to facilitate intubation?
4. Following the initial resuscitation, what X-rays are indicated?
5. What other intrathoracic injuries should be considered?

Discussion

This man has suffered a severe crush injury to the chest resulting in a clinically obvious left pneumothorax. The immediate priority in the resuscitation room is the relief of hypoxia, and the first step to be taken should be the insertion of an intercostal drain and connection to an underwater seal drain. This should be done by making a small incision under local anaesthesia; then, using blunt dissection, cutting down to the pleura and inserting the drain under direct vision (trochar type devices are potentially hazardous and should now be confined to the museum). Prior X-ray confirmation of the pneumothorax is not necessary and may even result in hazardous delay: X-ray departments are dangerous places! This patient will have extensive lung contusion and intra-alveolar haemorrhage; this will result in a considerable intrapulmonary shunt and blood loss, and a chest drain alone may well not relieve his hypoxaemia. The high blood pressure may mask considerable hypovolaemia; a large-bore (preferably 2) intravenous cannula should be inserted, and volume replacement commenced initially with a synthetic colloid solution such as Haemaccel or Gelofusine; these have a relatively short circulatory half-life but provide efficient initial volume expansion and allow 'room' for blood to be given later, when available.

The sensory level at D12 suggests a denervating injury (probably due to a burst fracture of a lower thoracic vertebra). However, at this early stage the use of suxamethonium is not precluded and indeed it would be positively indicated in view of the possibility of a full stomach and post-traumatic ileus. The presence of a level at D12 does not exclude the fact that there may be a coexisting, undiagnosed neck injury; the neck should therefore be immobilized in a stiff cervical collar, and sandbags placed on either side of the neck to maintain the head in a neutral position. It is probably true to say that minor degrees of movement associated with intubation will not result in any further deterioration in an unstable neck over and above that caused by the initial trauma. If it is felt clinically that particular difficulty might be encountered with intubation, then consideration should be given to a tracheostomy under local anaesthesia or a cricothyroidotomy, depending on the urgency of the situation.

Following the initial resuscitation, the radiographs likely to be of immediate value in the assessment of the patient are views of the chest, lateral cervical spine and (possibly) pelvis. All victims of major trauma should be assumed to have an unstable neck injury until proved otherwise, and managed accordingly with a *stiff* collar.

Persistent bubbling of the chest drain and the development of subcutaneous emphysema suggests the possibility of rupture of a main bronchus and this needs to be excluded by bronchoscopy. The patient should be transferred to theatre with the chest drain unclamped. If the patient had not been intubated, classic teaching would advise induction of anaesthesia with the patient breathing spontaneously and avoidance of the use of muscle relaxants. However, this can be technically difficult and may predispose to regurgitation. With a thoracic surgeon standing by it is acceptable to give the patient an intravenous induction agent followed by suxamethonium and permit the surgeon to pass the bronchoscope.

The side arm of the bronchoscope is then connected to a high-pressure oxygen outlet and the patient intermittently ventilated by means of a Sander's injector (Venturi principle), maintaining anaesthesia with increments of induction agent and suxamethonium (pretreatment with atropine or perhaps glycopyrronium). Should it prove impossible to ventilate the patient, it should be possible to pass a right-sided double lumen endobronchial tube, isolate the right lung and differentially ventilate while proceeding to thoracotomy.

Following initial resuscitative measures and securing the airway, a full and systematic examination of all trauma patients should be undertaken. Following a crush injury of sufficient force to result in a flail segment in a young man, a high index of suspicion should be held for other intrathoracic injuries, particularly pulmonary and myocardial contusion. Cardiac tamponade is more likely to result from penetrating injuries, whereas aortic tears are more likely to result from deceleration injuries. However, any suspicion of a widened mediastinum should lead to early arteriography.

Case 9

A 72-year-old man was admitted to the intensive care unit following a laparotomy for faecal peritonitis due to a perforated diverticulum. A Hartmann's procedure was performed and he was subsequently transferred to the intensive care unit for overnight ventilation. After 6 hours, however, his condition deteriorated.

The patient was found to be febrile with a temperature of 39°C and a tachycardia of 130 beats/min; the blood pressure had fallen from 130/80 mmHg to 90/40 mmHg. Clinically he appeared warm and well perfused, but the urine output had fallen from 60 ml to 15 ml per hour. Arterial blood gases had deteriorated:

Mechanically ventilated: Fio_2 0.6, pH 7.28, Po_2 8.1 mmHg, Pco_2 4.8 mmHg, base deficit -10 mmol/l

Full blood count values were haemoglobin 9.8 g/dl, white cell count 16.7×10^9/l and platelets 58×10^9/l. The chest X-ray is shown in *Figure 9a*.

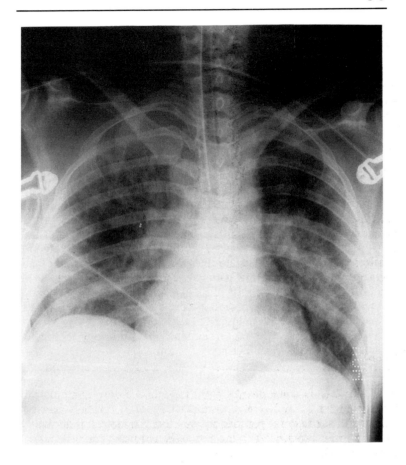

Figure 9a

Questions

1. What is the likely cause of the deterioration?
2. What are the possible mechanisms involved in this process?
3. What further monitoring would you require to manage this patient optimally? What are the major risks?
4. How would you calculate the systemic vascular resistance? Calculate the value at step 1 (*Table 9a*). How are the units arrived at? (Assume 1 atmosphere pressure equals 760 mmHg,

Table 9a

	Step 1	Step 2	Step 3
Mean arterial pressure (mmHg)	54	60	70
Central venous pressure (mmHg)	12	16	10
Pulmonary artery occlusion pressure (mmHg)	5	14	11
Cardiac index (l/m^2)	2.5	2.8	3.9
Systemic vascular resistance ($dyn.s/cm^5$)	?	698	684

the density of mercury is 13.6 g/ml, the acceleration due to gravity is 981 cm/s^2 and the body surface area is 1.8 m^2.) Step 1 (*Table 9a*) shows the initial readings obtained. Indicate the appropriate treatment between steps 1 and 2, steps 2 and 3 and after step 3.

5. How would you calculate the oxygen delivery index and consuption index of the patient, assuming a cardiac output of 5 l/min, a haemoglobin level of 10 g/dl, arterial oxygen saturation of 95% and a mixed venous oxygen saturation of 70%, while neglecting the small amount of oxygen in solution?
6. What principles govern treatment? Is there any definitive treatment worth considering?

Discussion

This man has become profoundly shocked. The shock is probably septicaemic in nature, with the septic focus arising from the faecal peritonitis. The clinical picture is mediated by the initiation and interaction of a series of cascade mechanisms as yet not wholly understood, the final result of which is the liberation of a number of cytotoxic mediators leading to multiple organ failure. The intact intestinal mucosa usually provides an effective barrier to the absorption of lipopolysaccharide endotoxins. This protection appears to be lost in septicaemic states, perhaps due to hypoxia, reperfusion injury or the action of oxygen free radicals, and endotoxaemia results. Endotoxin is capable of activating a number of cascade mechanisms such as coagulation, fibrinolysis and complement activation; these result in a multitude of effects such as polymorph chemotaxis, free radical production and the activation of cellular components of immunity such as macrophages/monocytes, lymphocytes and endothelial cells. These cells release a number of cytotoxic mediators; the most important (certainly the most topical) is tumour necrosis factor, produced by macrophages. Interactions occur with other important cytokines such as interleukin I, platelet activating factor from endothelial cells and leucocytes, whilst activated polymorphs release damage mediators such as oxygen free radicals, proteinases and phospholipid-derived products such as thromboxane and the leukotrienes. The permeability of endothelial cells is increased and a capillary leak syndrome develops. Disseminated intravascular coagulation is triggered by the production of procoagulant tissue factors. The resulting fibrin production causes separation of endothelial cells, disruption of the microcirculation and increases in the systemic and pulmonary vascular permeability.

For his optimal treatment this patient requires a flow-directed pulmonary artery catheter in order that filling pressures in the left side of the heart can be known and acted upon, thus permitting the optimal use of inotropes and/or vasoconstrictors in the treatment of the hypotension. The major risks are those of central venous line insertion plus the production of arrhythmias when crossing the tricuspid valve, sepsis, pulmonary infarction, pulmonary artery rupture and air embolism if the balloon bursts (particularly hazardous in the presence of intracardiac right to left shunts, when a case can be made for inflating the balloon with carbon dioxide). To obtain useful clinical data, the siting of the Swan-Ganz catheter should meet certain criteria. The wedge trace should resemble an atrial waveform with an 'a' and a 'v' wave, and have a lower value than the pulmonary artery diastolic pressure. In equating the pulmonary artery occlusion pressure with the left ventricular end-diastolic pressure it is assumed that there is a continuous column of blood with no flow between the occluded branch of the pulmonary artery and the left ventricle with the mitral valve open. It should thus be possible to aspirate blood with a high P_{O_2} from the catheter when it is said to lie within a West's zone III position, i.e. where the pulmonary artery pressure exceeds the pulmonary venous pressure, which in turn exceeds the alveolar pressure.

The systemic vascular resistance (SVR) is given by

$$SVR = (MAP - RAP)/CO$$

Where MAP is the mean arterial pressure, RAP is the right atrial pressure (central venous pressure) and CO is the cardiac output. The units of systemic vascular resistance are $dyn.s/cm^5$; we therefore need to convert the blood pressure, traditionally measured in mmHg, into dyn/cm^2 (1 dyn is the force required to accelerate 1 g by 1 cm/s/s).

The force F required to support a column of mercury 76 cm high is given by the equation

$$F = \text{depth} \times \text{density} \times \text{acceleration due to gravity} \times \text{area}$$

Expressed in terms of units:

$$F = \text{cm} \times (\text{g/cm}^3) \times (\text{cm/s}^2) \times \text{cm}^2$$
$$= \text{g.cm/s}^2 \text{ or dyn}$$

Therefore force per unit area

$$= 76 \times 13.6 \times 981 = 1.014 \times 10^6 \text{ dyn/cm}^2$$

Therefore

$$1 \text{ mmHg} = 1.014 \times 10^6/760 = 1334 \text{ dyn/cm}^2$$

The cardiac output is the product of the cardiac index and the body surface area. For step 1

$$\text{CO} = 2.5 \times 1.8 = 4.5 \text{ l/min} = 75 \text{ ml/s}$$

The systemic vascular resistance can thus be calculated as follows:

$$\text{SVR} = (\text{MAP} - \text{RAP})/\text{CO} = 1334 \times (54 - 12)/75$$
$$= 747 \text{ dyn.s/cm}^5$$

SVR may be rapidly calculated from:

$$\text{SVR} = \frac{\text{MAP} - \text{RAP}}{\text{CO}} \times 80$$

The first set of haemodynamic variables suggests that the patient has a low left atrial pressure as reflected by the pulmonary artery occlusion pressure (PAOP, or frequently in common parlance the 'wedge') and that left ventricular performance could be improved by volume expansion. In effect this reading suggests that taken in conjunction with his arterial gases and the radiological appearance, the patient is exhibiting the 'low pressure' pulmonary oedema of the 'adult respiratory distress syndrome, (or acute lung injury). Blood transfusion would be appropriate to aim at a haemoglobin level of around 12–13 g/dl or, if blood is not available, a colloid solution, preferably one with large molecules such as hetastarch or human albumin solution that will favour retention within the intravascular space and be less likely to cross 'leaky' capillaries. There is, however, little response in terms of cardiac output and blood pressure despite an adequate PAOP at step 2, and the next step would be the addition of an inotrope such as dobutamine. Although this increases cardiac output at step 3, the patient remains hypotensive due to vasodilatation, a feature characteristic of septic shock (normal range of SVR 770–1500 dyn.s/cm^5), and treatment of the hypotension with a vasoconstrictor such as noradrenaline would be appropriate.

The oxygen availability D_{O_2} is the product of arterial oxygen content and cardiac output; neglecting the oxygen carried in simple solution, it is given by:

$$D_{O_2} = Q \times (\text{Hb} \times 1.34 \times \%\ O_2\ \text{saturation})$$

Where Q is the cardiac output, Hb is the haemoglobin concentration in g/dl and 1.34 is the volume of oxygen in ml carried by 1 g of haemoglobin. For this patient,

$$\begin{aligned} D_{O_2} &= 5000 \times (10 \times 1.34 \times 0.95)/100 \\ &= 636.5\ \text{ml/min} \\ &= 353.6\ \text{ml/min/m}^2 \end{aligned}$$

(It is necessary to divide by 100 as the cardiac output is in ml/min and the Hb value is g per dl, i.e. 100 ml.)

Similarly, the oxygen consumption is obtained by calculating the mixed venous oxygen content using a pulmonary artery sample whose haemoglobin saturation must be measured directly using an oximeter (i.e. not derived from the assumed curve of a blood gas analyser) and subtracting from the oxygen availability calculated above.

$$\begin{aligned} \text{Mixed venous } O_2 \text{ content} &= 10 \times 1.34 \times 0.7 \\ &= 9.38\ \text{ml per 100 ml blood} \\ \text{Arterial } O_2 \text{ content} &= 10 \times 1.34 \times 0.95 \\ &= 12.73\ \text{ml per 100 ml blood} \end{aligned}$$

Therefore

$$\begin{aligned} \text{arterio-venous difference} &= 12.73 - 9.38 \\ &= 3.35\ \text{ml per 100 ml blood} \end{aligned}$$

As the cardic output is 5000 ml/min

$$\text{Oxygen consumption } V_{O_2} = (3.35 \times 5000)/100$$
$$= 167.5 \text{ ml/min}$$

Dividing by the body surface area gives the oxygen consumption index:

$$= 167.5/1.8 = 93 \text{ ml/min/m}^2$$

The rationale for treatment of septic shock states lies in physiological support of the failing organ system by endeavouring to optimize oxygen delivery to the tissues. These patients frequently exhibit a tissue oxygen debt, characterized by an elevated blood lactate level due to ongoing anaerobic metabolism at tissue level. There is evidence that survival may be improved in these patients by optimizing mean arterial presure, cardiac index and oxygen delivery and consumption (D_{O_2} and V_{O_2}). Success should be reflected by a fall in the lactate level. These patients frequently demonstrate the phenomenon of supply-dependent oxygen consumption. The presence of supply dependency may be demonstrated by means of a dobutamine challenge where a patient (who has received adequate volume resuscitation to an appropriate pulmonary artery occlusion pressure) is administered a dose of dobutamine to increase the cardiac output and thus the oxygen delivery. If supply dependency is present there should be an increase in the V_{O_2}, no change or a fall in the mixed venous oxygen saturation or an improvement in the blood lactate concentration. Conversely, a constant extraction of oxygen in the face of an increased cardiac output will be reflected by an increase in the mixed venous oxygen saturation. Pulmonary artery catheters are now available incorporating a probe employing the principle of reflectance oximetry to give continuous monitoring of the mixed venous oxygen saturation. Optimal 'goals' have been suggested by Shoemaker and others (CI 4.5l/min./m^2, D_{O_2} 600 ml/min./m^2 and V_{O_2} 170 ml/min./m^2). Nevertheless, the blind use of large doses of inotropes without evidence of supply dependency is not without its hazards, particularly in terms of the balance between myocardial oxygen supply and demand.

Of recent interest is the development of an IgM human monoclonal antibody to the lipid A moiety of endotoxin. A recent multicentre trial has demonstrated a significantly improved survival in patients with proven gram negative septicaemia. The patient in this case would certainly meet most recognized entry criteria for the use of this drug—fever, tachycardia and ventilator dependency along with signs of systemic toxicity such as acidosis, hypotension with a low systemic vascular resistance, a falling platelet count and possibly impending acute renal failure. Serious consideration should be given to administering a single 100 mg intravenous dose.

Case 10

A 45-year-old Scottish woman was scheduled for a routine arthroscopy. She was generally fit and well, but after an anaesthetic some 10 years ago she developed severe vomiting and abdominal pain associated with some weakness and mental confusion. This resolved over the ensuing 2 weeks. The notes relating to this previous anaesthetic were unavailable.

A full blood count revealed a haemoglobin level of 11.2 g/dl, a white cell count of 8.2×10^9/l and a platelet count of 305×10^9/l. The ECG is shown in *Figure 10a*.

Questions

1. What does the ECG show? Explain the appearance in electrical terms. Do you think it is relevant to the conduct of this anaesthetic?
2. What do you think happened 10 years ago?
3. Explain the pathophysiology underlying this patient's condition. How would you confirm your suspicions?
4. How would this influence the conduct of the anaesthesia on this occasion?

Discussion

This woman's ECG shows right bundle branch block (RBBB). The QRS complex shows the characteristic RSR' configuration and the QR interval is greater than 0.12 seconds. In a fit patient with no other cardiovascular symptomatology this is generally regarded as an isolated finding with no adverse implications, although it may be associated with pulmonary hypertension, right heart strain, etc.

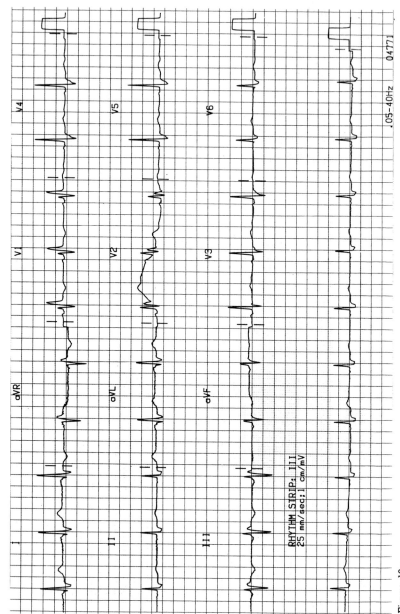

Figure 10a

In the normal heart the interventricular septum is depolarized first from left to right; thus a lead such as V_1 or V_2, looking at the right ventricle, will record an initial upward deflection (R wave). This is followed by synchronous depolarization of the left and right ventricles, which will appear as a downward deflection; this is because the greater muscle mass of the left ventricle makes the greater contribution to the net voltage, which will thus be negative with respect to a lead oriented towards the right side of the heart. In RBBB the right main bundle is blocked and there is delayed, retrograde depolarization of the right ventricle occurring after left ventricular depolarization; this is detected as the second, delayed R′ deflection.

This patient's previous exposure to surgery and anaesthesia was complicated by an attack of porphyria, which in a Scottish woman was almost certainly of the acute intermittent variety.

The porphyrias are a group of congenitally acquired metabolic defects in the synthetic pathway for haem. The porphyrins are intermediate compounds in haem synthesis. The key point in the synthetic pathway is the activity of the enzyme aminolaevulinic acid (ALA) synthetase. Haem itself normally acts as the negative feedback of this enzyme but its activity may be stimulated by a number of drugs and pathophysiological states.

Acute intermittent porphyria (AIP) is an autosomal dominant condition due to reduced activity of an enzyme early in the haem synthetic pathway; uroporphyrinogen I synthetase. Surprisingly, perhaps, anaemia is not a feature of the condition, but the resulting overactivity of ALA synthetase leads to a build-up of intermediate porphyrins prior to the enzymatic block. These porphyrins (namely δ-aminolaevulinic acid and porphobilinogen) are smaller molecules than those occurring later on in the synthetic chain and are able to gain access to the cerebral cortex, with resulting neuropsychiatric symptoms. In the other two relatively common porphyric states — variegate porphyria and porphyria cutanea tarda — the metabolic block occurs later in the chain, leading to overproduction of higher molecular weight porphyrins. These are relatively excluded from the central nervous system, but collect in the skin, where they cause the well-recognized photosensitivity when irradiated with ultraviolet light.

In AIP the diagnosis is confirmed by the detection of raised levels of ALA and porphobilinogen in the urine.

Optimal anaesthetic technique lies in avoiding drugs that are known to precipitate attacks by increasing the activity of ALA synthetase. Remember, adverse physiological states such as hypoglycaemia and dehydration will also have this effect. The most important agents to avoid are thiopentone and other barbiturates such as methohexitone. Etomidate has been shown to increase ALA synthetase activity in vitro, and propofol has been shown to result in increased urinary porphyrin excretion, but both have been used clinically without adverse sequelae. The opiates appear safe along with nitrous oxide and the volatile agents, although there is a question mark over halothane. All the relaxants (with the possible exception of pancuronium) are safe. The picture is less clear with regard to the benzodiazepines, but diazepam has a record of safety in the condition. This particular operation could well be performed under a regional block; bupivacaine has been shown to be safe, whilst lignocaine, porphyrinogenic in the rat, has been used uneventfully in humans.

Peroperatively, 10% dextrose should probably be given to prevent precipitating an attack from hypoglycaemia, and there should be meticulous avoidance of dehydration.

Case 11

A 22-year-old black man had been chronically unwell since the age of 6 months. He suffered recurrent pneumonias and intermittent episodes of severe abdominal pain. He had developed gallstones and now required a cholecystectomy.

Features noted on examination were pale conjunctivae, slight jaundice and a healing ulcer on the left leg. The pulse was regular at 105 beats/min, the blood pressure was 130/80 mmHg, and first and second heart sounds were noted. The patient's chest was clear, and the urine was of normal colour. Results of laboratory investigations were haemoglobin 7.0 g/dl, white cell count $14.5 \times 10^9/l$, platelets $350 \times 10^9/l$, packed cell volume 20% and reticulocytes 18%. Liver function tests gave the following values: bilirubin 50 μmol/l, AST normal, alkaline phosphatase normal.

Questions

1. What is the nature of the anaemia?
2. What is the most likely explanation for the jaundice?

3. Explain the clinical findings in terms of the underlying disease. Why did symptoms commence at 6 months of age? How are exacerbations provoked?
4. How should the diagnosis be cofirmed?
5. How should the patient be prepared preoperatively? Would you think bicarbonate therapy a useful manoeuvre? Would you transfuse blood preoperatively?
6. Are any special precautions necessary preoperatively?

Discussion

This young man has a haemolytic anaemia with a low haemoglobin level, reticulocytosis and a modest elevation of the serum bilirubin. In this clinical situation jaundice could be caused either by an unconjugated hyperbilirubinaemia due to haemolysis, where haem breakdown exceeds the capacity of the liver to conjugate the bilirubin, or by an obstructive jaundice due to stones in the common bile duct resulting in conjugated hyperbilirubinaemia. Haemolysis is the cause in this case. If the patient had been suffering from obstructive jaundice the urine would be darkened due to the presence of the water-soluble conjugated bilirubin, and the alkaline phosphatase would probably be elevated.

In a black patient the cause of this haemolytic anaemia is almost certainly sickle-cell disease. This is the result of an abnormal amino acid substitution on the beta chain of the haemoglobin molecule (valine substituted for glutamic acid at the 6 position on the chain). When exposed to a lowered Po_2 red cells containing this abnormal haemoglobin undergo a reversible change in shape from the normal biconcave disc to an irregular form; this is brought about by an intracellular polymerization reaction which is initiated when the haemoglobin saturation is around 85% (corresponding to a Po_2 in the range of 40–50 mmHg) and is complete at around 38% saturation. The implication is that a sickle-cell patient with a normal venous oxygen saturation of around 75% is in a chronic state of haemolysis.

The patient is chronically unwell due to anaemia but the course is punctuated by frequent infections and ischaemic crises due to vaso-occlusion of the microcirculation by clumps of sickle cells. This results in splenic sequestration, which accounts for the attacks of abdominal pain, leg ulcers, avascular necrosis of bone and pulmonary infarcts ultimately leading to pulmonary hypertension. Aplastic as well as haemolytic crises can occur and patients are at risk of chronic infection and overwhelming sepsis. Prophylactic antibiotics and pneumococcal vaccine are indicated throughout childhood. The hyperbilirubinaemia results in the formation of gallstones which are a common reason for surgical intervention in these patients at a relatively young age.

Crises may be precipitated by acidosis, dehydration, cold, exertion, infection and vascular stasis, as well as by hypoxia.

The diagnosis should be confirmed by haemoglobin electrophoresis. Simple solubility tests for haemoglobin S may be unrealiable. Electrophoresis will also differentiate the disease from other forms such as sickle-cell trait (Hb-AS), Hb-SC disease and Hb-S thalassaemia.

Careful preparation is required prior to surgery. Prophylactic antibiotics should be given, and (if not already prescribed) folic acid supplements should be commenced. Dehydration may be countered by giving intravenous fluids during the starvation period, which in any case should not be prolonged. As acidosis promotes sickling it has been suggested that bicarbonate administration may be useful. However, the oxygen dissociation curve is favourably shifted to the right in sickle-cell anaemia to facilitate the unloading of oxygen at the tissues. Bicarbonate therapy would shift the curve to the left and negate this favourable adaptation.

The greatest area of controversy lies in the place of preoperative transfusion. Older series tended to favour the conservative use of blood transfusion bearing in mind the risks of alloimmunization, iron overload and the transmission of infection. However, more recent series suggest improved morbidity and mortality following the use of simple transfusion prior to minor surgery and exchange transfusion prior to major procedures. Approximate guidelines are to increase the haematocrit to around 30–35% and to reduce the percentage of Hb-S to less than 30, although controversy exists as to what the safe level of Hb-S might be.

There is no specific 'best technique' for these patients; more important is the care with which the chosen technique is performed. Preoxygenation is a sensible precaution, as is the extended use of oxygen in the postoperative period to attenuate postoperative hypoxaemia. The contribution to hypoxaemia from reduced basal ventilation due to abdominal pain may be attenuated by good analgesia — perhaps the use of intercostal nerve blocks or even a thoracic epidural block. Cold may be minimized by the use of warming blankets, warmed intravenous fluids and the humidification of inspired gases. Pulse oximetry and capnography are valuable, and intra-arterial monitoring will permit frequent blood gas analysis to give early warning of any acidosis.

Although probably not relevant to a cholecystectomy, regional techniques using spinal and epidural blockade might be appropriate for other forms of surgery. Volume loading should be generous with the aim of avoiding the use of vasoconstrictor agents in the treatment of hypotension. Bier's block would be contraindicated due to vascular stasis and the build-up of a tissue acidosis which would be released into the circulation on cuff deflation. If tourniquets are required their use should be kept to an absolute minimum.

The signs of a peroperative sickle-cell crisis are harder to detect under general anaesthesia, particularly when relaxants are employed, and an index of suspicion should exist that any evidence of organ dysfunction may be due to a vaso-occlusive crisis; treatment with fresh blood should be given to reduce the percentage of Hb-S and antibiotics used to treat infection.

Case 12

A 52-year-old woman with long-standing Crohn's disease required a laparotomy for a further bowel resection. She kept reasonably well but tended to tire easily, was dyspnoeic with moderate effort, prone to ankle oedema and had a tendency to bruise easily.

On examination the patient was found to be pale, with mild jaundice, finger clubbing and spider naevi. The cardiovascular and respiratory systems were unremarkable. The abdomen showed moderate distension with shifting dullness; the liver was palpable 2 cm below the costal margin and the tip of the spleen was palpable. Laboratory investigations gave the following values:

Full blood count: haemoglobin 11.2 g/dl, white cell count $4.8 \times 10^9/l$, platelets $118 \times 10^9/l$
Coagulation screen: prothrombin ratio 1.5 × control
Urea and electrolytes: sodium 128 mmol/l, potassium 4.5 mmol/l, chloride 100 mmol/l, bicarbonate 28 mmol/l, urea 7.2 mmol/l
Creatinine 198 μmol/l
Liver function: bilirubin 45 μmol/l, albumin 26 g/l, AST 172 U/l (normal 5–42 U/l), alkaline phosphatase 700 U/l (normal 100–300 U/l)

46

1. What is the secondary pathology? Relate the results to the clinical picture. How do you palpate for an equivocal spleen, and what is the likely significance of the splenomegaly in this case?
2. Identify the major risks that this patient is likely to encounter with surgery and anaesthesia. What steps would you take to minimize these? Would you require any further investigations?
3. Which anaesthetic drug would you employ in giving this woman general anaesthesia?
4. If intraoperative bleeding failed to respond to fresh frozen plasma and platelets, what other agents might have a useful role to play?

Discussion

This patient has the symptoms and signs of chronic liver failure, and this finding is supported by the biochemical investigations. The aetiology when associated with long-standing Crohn's disease is likely to be sclerosing cholangitis. Clubbing is a feature of Crohn's disease and the spider naevi are thought to be the result of the diseased liver being unable to metabolize circulating oestrogens. It is important to appreciate that the normal liver has a large functional reserve and so evidence of liver failure only becomes apparent after considerable liver destruction has taken place. By asking the patient to roll towards the examiner it is possible to improve the chances of detecting splenomegaly, and its presence in this case suggests the presence of portal hypertension. The hypoalbuminaemia contributes to the formation of peripheral oedema, which, in association with the portal hypertension, contributes to the abdominal distension and the formation of ascites. The liver is responsible for the manufacture of all the clotting factors with the exception of factor VIII, and their reduced production results in the prolongation of the prothrombin time.

It is the functional reserve of the liver rather than the aetiology of the cirrhosis that is of greater importance to the anaesthetist. From the respiratory point of view, cirrhotic patients develop intrapulmonary shunts of obscure aetiology and there is impairment of hypoxic pulmonary vasoconstriction. Preoperative blood gas analysis would therefore be valuable. A chest X-ray is also indicated in this situation to exclude pleural effusions. Significant ascites will cause splinting of the diaphragm, and coupled with the pain following abdominal surgery could result in a considerable fall in the functional residual capacity, basal atelectasis and hypoxia. Epidural anaesthesia would be contraindicated owing to the presence of a coagulopathy.

Renal function should be evaluated preoperatively because the hepatorenal syndrome is particularly likely to develop in this group. Postoperative renal failure in this situation carries a high mortality.

Not only is there reduced clotting factor production in liver failure but increased fibrinolysis also contributes to the coagulopathy. Coagulation should be normalized as far as possible preoperatively by giving vitamin K, to encourage the production of the vitamin K-dependent factors (II, VII, IX and X), fresh frozen plasma and platelets if necessary.

If not known, the hepatitis B status of the patient should be checked in view of the need for special precautions if it is positive.

No particular anaesthetic recipe exists for these patients. All surgery and anaesthesia will reduce liver blood flow and potentially decompensate the failing liver. In essence a technique appropriate for the surgery should be adopted, employing drugs that are not themselves hepatotoxic and which as far as possible do not rely on the liver for their elimination.

Oral premedication would be preferable to an intramuscular injection, and lorazepam is said to be preferable to diazepam for this purpose.

Induction may be safely achieved with a carefully titrated dose of thiopentone as initial recovery from the drug is due to redistribution, although the slow elimination phase due to hepatic metabolism may be prolonged.

Low levels of plasma cholinesterase mean a prolonged action of suxamethonium should be anticipated, but this should not matter clinically for surgery of reasonable duration. Atracurium is the relaxant of choice as its elimination via Hofmann degradation is independent of the liver. Fentanyl appears to be a satisfactorily handled analgesic and would probably be preferable to morphine which requires hepatic 6-glucuronidation for its metabolism. Hepatomegaly and splenomegaly lead to an increased blood flow to these organs, tending to necessitate larger and more frequent doses of non-depolarizing muscle relaxants to maintain a given level of neuromuscular blockade. This may be compounded in some types of cirrhosis where there are elevations in the levels of circulating globulins leading to increased protein binding. Iso-flurane would be the obvious choice of volatile agent as it undergoes minimal metabolism (0.2% compared with 2% for enflurane and 20% for halothane).

Peroperative renal protection is vital with the use of mannitol and 'renal' doses of dopamine. Meticulous fluid balance (prefe-rably under CVP control) is essential, with losses replaced volume for volume with allowance for evaporation. Protein loss from the abdominal cavity should be anticipated and countered with salt-poor albumin.

If persistent bleeding resistant to fresh frozen plasma and platelets is a problem, consideration should be given to agents that inhibit fibrinolysis, such as ε-aminocaproic acid and aprotinin. Platelet adhesion may be improved by the use of desmopressin (DDAVP).

Case 13

A woman of 40 visited her general practitioner complaining of pain in the left eye and double vision. He examined the eye, noted a dilated pupil, a divergent squint and ptosis, and referred her to a neurologist. While awaiting her appointment she collapsed with a severe occipital headache associated with photophobia and neck stiffness; she was drowsy but rousable, and had no focal neurolo-gical signs. This woman had a vague past history of dark-coloured urine in the morning and a deep venous thrombosis; it is known that she was investiated by a haematologist some years previously but did not attend for follow-up.

Laboratory investigation revealed a haemoglobin level of 11.1 g/dl, a white cell count of 2.3×10^9/l and a platelet count of 120×10^9/l.

Questions

1. What is described at this patient's initial presentation? How does it further the acute diagnosis? How would you confirm the acute diagnosis?

2. What are the chief considerations to be taken into account regarding the timing of operative intervention, and what prior investigations might be useful?
3. Are there any useful therapeutic interventions?
4. Although used less often, induced hypotension may be required for surgery in this condition. Indicate two ways this might be achieved.
5. What is the major consideration in the patient's postoperative care?
6. What do you think her chronic haematological condition might be? Does it impose any added risks, and how might these be countered?

Discussion

The patient presented to her general practitioner with a third nerve palsy. One well-recognized cause of an isolated third nerve palsy is an aneurysm of the posterior communicating artery. She subsequently presented with the signs and symptoms of a sub-arachnoid haemorrhage resulting from its rupture. This can be confirmed on lumbar puncture by the finding of blood and xanthochromia in the cerebrospinal fluid. Computed tomographic scanning, now increasingly available, is generally regarded as a safer way of securing the diagnosis.

Definitive surgical treatment requires the placing of a spring clip around the neck of the aneurysm. The initial bleed can result in vasospasm of the cerebral circulation and loss of normal autoregulatory capacity. Operation at this early stage carries a greater risk of impairment of cerebral blood flow, and subsequent damage, particularly if induced hypotension is contemplated. However, if surgery is delayed until the patient is in better condition, there is the ever-present risk of a catastrophic re-bleed during the waiting period. This remains an area of neurosurgical controversy, and in general it is the patient's condition that determines the timing of the operation.

Prior to surgery, efforts are directed towards establishing the site of the aneurysm (and looking for multiple aneurysms) with cerebral angiography, preventing further rupturing and relieving vasospasm. The chances of re-bleeding are increased if surges of hypertension are allowed to occur or the intracranial pressure is permitted to fall precipitously. Patients should be nursed in a quiet environment. Hypotensive agents should be used to treat severe hypertension, but blood pressure should not be lowered drastically as cerebral perfusion could drop to critical levels in the presence of vasospasm. Beta-blockers may be useful agents in this respect, bearing in mind that a significant minority of patients with a subarachnoid bleed have ECG evidence of ischaemia. Similarly, osmotic agents such as mannitol should be avoided. Cerebral angiography is necessary but hazardous; general anaesthesia is rarely employed but heavy sedation is appropriate. Antifibrinolytic agents such as tranexamic acid are sometimes used to retard clot breakdown, although there is little evidence of dramatic benefit. Recently nimodipine, a calcium antagonist, has shown some promise in the relief of vasospasm. With the advent of non-invasive techniques for the measurement of cerebral blood flow, it is now possible to test the autoregulatory capacity of the cerebral circulation by reducing the blood pressure with an agent such as trimetaphan and recording the changes in cerebral blood flow to see if it is still pressure-dependent or whether autoregulatory capacity has returned. This information may assist in the timing of surgery.

Induced hypotension used to be very popular in surgery for intracranial aneurysms, but it is increasingly recognized that it may be an important contributor to postoperative morbidity in the presence of vasospasm. Peroperative normotension and modest normocapnia are now the rule, and brief periods of induced hypotension are reserved for dissection close to large and technically difficult aneurysms. Sodium nitroprusside remains a popular direct-acting vasodilator with a rapid onset and offset of action; it is generally administered as a 0.01% solution, the chief problem being metabolic acidosis and cyanide toxicity which may result from prolonged high-dose infusions (total doses in excess of 50 mg). Glyceryl trinitrate is less popular as a hypotension-inducing agent in neurosurgery owing to its slower onset in action and longer termination of effect; it also has cerebral vasodilator properties. Isoflurane has become the volatile agent of choice in neurosurgery as it has a relatively small effect on cerebral blood flow and volume compared with the other volatile agents. Due to its effect of reducing blood pressure by a greater action on the systemic vascular resistance than on cardiac output, it is a useful agent for providing controlled hypotension in neurosurgery. It is more difficult to induce hypotension if hypercarbia is allowed to develop, and in younger, fitter patients.

The major postoperative problem is the development of cerebral ischaemia due to vasospasm. Once the aneurysm is safely clipped it is safe to try to overcome this by maintaining the patient in a slightly hyperhydrated state with a mean arterial pressure of 120–130 mmHg (assuming normotension at the outset). This may be achieved with alternate administration of colloid and crystalloid at volumes of 3–4 litres per day.

This woman's chronic haematological condition is paroxysmal nocturnal haemoglobinuria. In its mild form it may only amount to occasional episodes of haemolysis at night, but these patients may develop aplastic crises and the condition may be preleukaemic. Subjects are prone to an increased incidence of venous thrombosis. It is arguable whether prophylaxis would be advisable here. Certainly prior to clipping, the risks of a re-bleed vastly outweigh the risks of deep venous thrombosis, and heparin would also be contraindicated following intracranial surgery. In general, intracranial surgery is not high for postoperative thrombogenic problems, but in this case some form of mechanical prophylaxis such as inflatable trousers may be worth considering.

Case 14

A 26-year-old vagrant was admitted unconscious and noted to be hyperventilating. No history was available.

On examination the man was found to have a regular pulse of 115 beats/min and blood pressure of 130/80 mmHg. First and second heart sounds were normal, and he was clinically warm and well perfused. There was marked hyperventilation, the chest was clear clinically and there were no focal neurological signs. Laboratory investigations gave the following values:

Full blood count: haemoglobin 14.8 g/dl, white cell count 22×10^9/l, platelets 290×10^9/l

Urea and electrolytes: sodium 135 mmol/l, potassium 5.0 mmol/l, chloride 100 mmol/l, bicarbonate 5 mmol/l, urea 7 mmol/l, glucose 5 mmol/l

Arterial blood gases (air): pH 6.9, P_{O_2} 11.5 kPa, P_{CO_2} 1.8 kPa, base deficit -24 mmol/l

Serum calcium 2.05 mmol/l, albumin 40 g/l
Serum osmolality 330 mosmol/kg/H$_2$0

The ECG is shown in *Figure 14a*.

Questions

1. What is the primary metabolic abnormality?
2. Explain how the other measurements strongly suggest a diagnosis. What is the likely diagnosis?
3. What are the three most important steps in the management of this patient? Explain the rationale behind them.
4. After a full recovery this man gives a history of intermittent episodes of rapid palpitation. Can you identify the cause?

Discussion

This patient has a severe metabolic acidosis with a large base deficit. He is attempting to compensate for this by lowering the carbon dioxide tension through hyperventilation.

$$CO_2 + H_2O \rightleftharpoons H_2CO_3 \rightleftharpoons HCO_3^- + H^+$$

The clue to the diagnosis lies in the increased 'anion gap' and the increased osmolar gap. The so-called anion gap refers to the difference between the routinely measured cations (Na^+, K^+) and the routinely measured anions (Cl^-, HCO_3^-), and is usually around 16 mmol/l. There is no *true* anion gap as the sums of total positive and negative charges in the blood are equal; the difference is accounted for chiefly by albumin and some other small molecular ions. In a metabolic acidosis the bicarbonate level falls and if this is associated with a normal anion gap there will be a compensatory rise in the chloride concentration. In this case metabolic acidosis has occurred with a normal chloride value and an increased anion gap (35 mmol/l). This suggests the retention of non-volatile organic acids and implies renal failure, ketoacidosis, lactic acidosis or the ingestion of toxins. In this case the near-normal urea, normal glucose concentration and good circulatory condition strongly suggest the ingestion of a toxin.

In healthy patients the plasma osmolality can be estimated from:

$$2 \text{ (sodium)} + \text{ (urea)} + \text{ (glucose)}$$

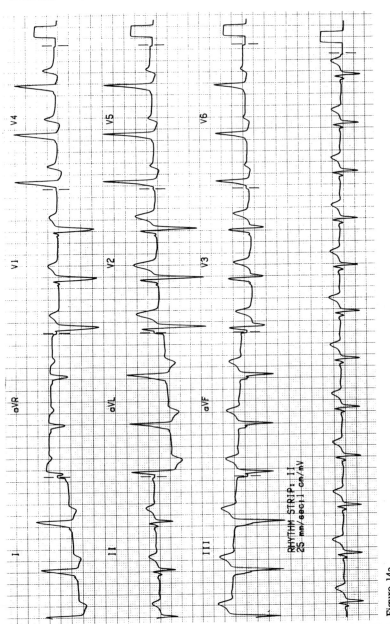

Figure 14a

The gap between this and the osmolality measured by freezing point depression should be less than $10\,mosmol/kgH_2O$, and is accounted for by calcium, lipids and proteins. In this case the calculated osmolality would be $282\,mosmol/kgH_2O$, giving an osmol gap of $48\,mosmol/kgH_2O$. As the osmolality of a solution is proportional to the molar concentrations of the osmotically active particles, the high osmol gap indicates the presence of a substance in high molar concentration (i.e. of relatively low molecular weight). Most drugs, including the salicylates, are large molecules and cannot attain sufficiently high molar concentrations to be identified in this way. Taken together, these findings form the picture of ethylene glycol intoxication. The hypocalcaemia and the leucocytosis are secondary clues. It is also worthwhile looking at the urine for oxaluria.

Ethylene glycol per se is relatively non-toxic; however, its highly acidic metabolites (chiefly glycolate and oxalate) are extremely toxic. Not only do they produce a severe metabolic acidosis, but they also cause central nervous system (CNS) toxicity and acute renal and cardiopulmonary failure. Approximately 100 ml may be lethal, with widespread deposition of oxalate crystals demonstrable throughout the CNS at postmortem. The metaboic acidosis must be treated vigorously and this may require large volumes of sodium bicarbonate (often 500–1000 ml of 8.4% $NaHCO_3$). Treatment of the acidosis is important not only for its own sake but also because low pH will favour the non-ionized, lipid-soluble moieties of the acidic metabolites, facilitating their access to the CNS via lipid-soluble membranes.

Ethylene glycol is rapidly metabolized in the liver by alcohol dehydrogenase; this offers the therapeutic potential of saturating the enzyme by the concomitant administration of alcohol. Following a loading dose (around 60 g in an adult) ethanol can be infused to retard the metabolism of the ethylene glycol, adjusting the infusion to achieve a serum ethanol concentration of around 15 mmol/l. However, the volume of distribution of ethylene glycol approximates to the total body water (0.70 l/kg), and endogenous excretion via the kidney is slow. This necessitates the urgent establishment of haemodialysis to achieve rapid ethylene glycol removal, the bicarbonate and ethanol treatment effectively 'buying time' while this is established. The dialysis will also negate the problems of the sodium load consequent upon the large administration of bicarbonate. Bear in mind also that the rate of ethanol infusion will have to be increased to cover the ethanol removed by dialysis.

This man's episodes of palpitation are explained by his 12-lead ECG (*Figure 14a*). This shows the characteristic slurred delta wave at the beginning of the QRS complex associated with a short PR interval, characteristic of the Wolff–Parkinson–White syndrome. Aberrant conduction tissue results in episodes of re-entrant tachycardia manifesting as episodes of supraventricular tachycardia.

Case 15

A 70-year-old man with long-standing hypertension developed acute chest pain radiating through to the back.

On examination the patient was found to be in pain; his pulse was regular at 80 beats/min, absent in the left hand, and his blood pressure was 200/120 mmHg. First and second heart sounds were heard, with a loud S_2. The chest was clear. Blood testing gave normal results for a full blood count and for urea and electrolytes. The ECG is shown in *Figure 15a* and the chest X-ray in *Figure 15b*.

Questions

1. What is the probable diagnosis?
2. What does the ECG show?
3. What treatment should be instituted while awaiting surgery or during transfer to a regional cardiothoracic centre?
4. What is the surgical approach? How can the anaesthetist facilitate surgical access? What tube would you use and what problems might be encountered?
5. If the procedure is successful, what is the major postoperative risk and what step could be taken peroperatively to avoid this?

Discussion

This man's ECG illustrates left ventricular hypertrophy with strain and is compatible with long-standing hypertension. The electrocardiographic criteria of left ventricular hypertrophy are met when the sum of the S wave in V_1 plus the R wave in V_5 — or

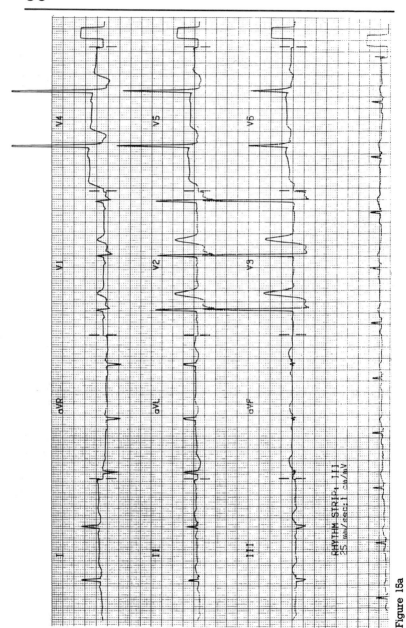

Figure 15a

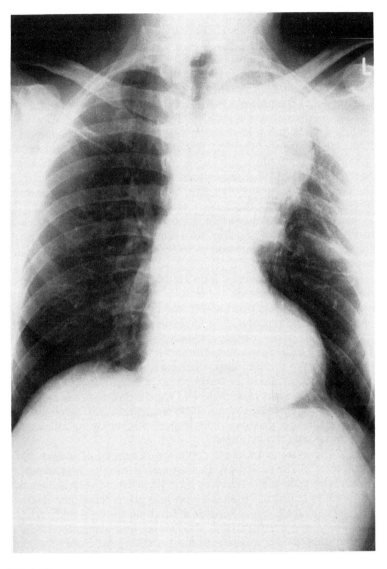

Figure 15b

alternatively S (V_2) plus R (V_6) — exceeds 35 mm. The ST segment depression in the lateral chest leads (the so-called strain pattern) is indicative of subendocardial ischaemia. However, there is no evidence of acute myocardial infarction to account for this man's sudden onset of chest pain.

The probable diagnosis is that he has suffered a dissection of the thoracic aorta. The loss of the radial pulse in the left hand suggests that the origin of the dissection is proximal to the origin of the left subclavian artery. Pathologically this is generally due to a transverse intimal tear, typically 5–6 cm above the aortic valve. It is clearly a very unstable situation and initial treatment is aimed at limiting the extent of the tear. Forward dissection may fortuitously dissect back into the aortic lumen resulting in the classic 'double-barrelled' aorta. More seriously, backward dissection may disrupt the aortic valve, involve the origin of the coronary arteries or open into the pericardium resulting in tamponade. Urgent angiography is indicated to delineate the extent of the tear. While this is awaited, or during transfer to a regional centre, hypotensive treatment should be initiated to keep the systolic blood pressure around 100 mmHg.

The surgical approach will be via a left thoracotomy. In order to improve surgical access a double lumen endobronchial tube should be passed so that the left lung may be collapsed out of the surgeon's way, and one lung anaesthesia continued via the right lung. This is most readily achieved by passing a right-sided Robertshaw tube. Some anaesthetists would argue that a left-sided tube should be passed, as greater care is required in placing the right-sided tube due to the early origin of the upper lobe bronchus from the right main bronchus. The right-sided tube always has a side hole for the right upper lobe bronchus, and care must be taken to ensure that the right upper lobe is being inflated by listening above the clavicles.

It is important to be clear about the sequence of events when siting one of these tubes. Passage is generally facilitated by turning the subject's head away from the side of the bronchus that you wish to intubate. When the tube is in place, inflate the tracheal cuff and ensure there is no leak around the tracheal cuff and that both lungs are inflating. Next, disconnect and clamp the tracheal inlet and check for inflation of the right lung (and only the right lung) via the bronchial inlet. Inflate the bronchial cuff. A leak will be heard by listening over the disconnected tracheal part of the tube; when the leak is abolished the bronchial cuff is sufficiently inflated. It is very easy to overinflate and risk herniation of the bronchial cuff. Finally disconnect and clamp the bronchial tube and inflate the tracheal portion, ensuring that the left lung inflates. Failure to inflate the left side and difficulty with inflation suggest that the tracheal opening is in the right main bronchus.

The major consideration during one lung anaesthesia (OLA) is to ensure adequate oxygenation is maintained, as the deflated lung will still take a considerable proportion of the pulmonary blood flow resulting in increased V/Q mismatching or shunt. Somewhat paradoxically, the better the function of the lung to be deflated the greater the problem is likely to be on OLA; for instance in empyema surgery, letting down a diseased lung which has formerly played little part in gas exchange will have little effect in increasing the shunt. One lung anaesthesia effectively halves the compliance of the lungs as a whole: tidal volumes will need to be reduced to prevent excessive inflation pressures and the frequency of ventilation increased to maintain the minute volume. Excess inflation pressures will merely increase the physiological dead space by collapsing pulmonary vessels.

It is traditional to increase the inspired oxygen concentration to 50% during OLA, but the routine availability of pulse oximetry allows the Fio_2 to be titrated against arterial saturations. Remember that volatile agents, even at low concentrations, impair the effect of hypoxic pulmonary vasoconstriction in the collapsed lung and will tend to aggravate the hypoxaemia. The use of volatile agents, however, is not generally contraindicated; indeed, their high potency permits the use of high inspired oxygen concentrations and they have favourable effects on bronchomotor tone. However, if hypoxaemia remains a problem, switching to an intravenous agent should be considered. Applying positive end-expiratory pressure (PEEP) to the dependent lung may also be helpful. Prior to closure of the chest the deflated lung should be adequately sucked out and inflation ensured.

One of the greatest hazards of operating on the thoracic aorta is the possibility of producing paraplegia by interrupting the blood supply to the anterior region of the spinal cord. This is derived from the artery of Adamkiewicz which has a variable origin from the thoracic aorta. It may be useful to continue the blood supply below the level of the aortic cross-clamp during surgery. This could be achieved by instituting normothermic left atriofemoral or femorofemoral bypass. The perfusionist then 'balances' the two circulations, drawing around 1 litre a minute from the left atrial return and allowing the remainder to pass to the left ventricle to perfuse the body above the aortic cross-clamp, and titrating the bypass flow against the arterial pressure (the arterial cannula would have to be in the right radial or brachial artery in this particular case).

Case 16

A fit 25-year-old woman with no previous record of exposure to anaesthesia presented for surgery to her varicose veins. Preoperative assessment was totally unremarkable and she was premedicated with papaveretum* and atropine. She was preoxygenated for 5 minutes, induced with thiopentone 300 mg, given suxamethonium 100 mg, intubated and allowed to breathe spontaneously. Anaesthesia was to be maintained with a mixture of 33% oxygen in 67% nitrous oxide supplemented with 2% halothane via a Bain circuit, with the fresh gas flow set at 9 l/min. The patient was transferred from the anaesthetic room to theatre and an ECG was connected which revealed a tachycardia of 150 beats/min. She was also thought to be sweating and mildly cyanosed. A pulse oximeter was attached which gave a reading of 83%.

Questions

1. What is your immediate reaction? What is the differential diagnosis?
2. If human error and equipment failures are excluded, what other clinical features might you expect to develop?
3. What is the underlying pathophysiology?
4. How would you manage the situation acutely?
5. How should the patient subsequently be investigated?
6. How would you anaesthetize her when (or if) she comes back for varicose vein surgery?

Discussion

The first consideration in this potentially catastrophic situation must be that a simple human or machine error has occurred, the most important being accidental intubation of the oesophagus. Marked cyanosis is not necessarily an early feature particularly if the patient has been well preoxygenated (a hazard of preoxygenation!). The only guaranteed way of ensuring that the endotracheal tube is in the trachea is to demonstrate carbon dioxide elimination by means of a capnograph. If there is the slightest doubt about the position of the tube it should be removed and the patient ventilated by hand with 100% oxygen (*if in doubt, take it out*).

Other possibilities to be excluded are that the patient has become disconnected from the anaesthetic machine or that an inadequate inspired oxygen concentration, as measured by an in-line oxygen analyser, is being delivered. Another possibility is that the patient is receiving extraneous carbon dioxide; check if the machine CO_2 rotameter has been left fully on, delivering 2 l/min. The Association of Anaesthetists now recommends that a cylinder of carbon dioxide should only be attached to the machine when it is actually required and removed when not actively in use. Another possibility in this case related to carbon dioxide accumulation is that the Bain circuit may not have been properly checked beforehand; a leak in the internal hose would result in massive rebreathing. Bain circuits (incidentally not an efficient choice in the spontaneously breathing patient) should be tested specifically for the integrity of the internal limb delivering the fresh gas flow by occluding it with the point of a pencil or similar object.

If equipment and human errors of this type are rapidly excluded it must be seriously considered that this patient is developing the malignant hyperpyrexia (MHP) syndrome. It is important to appreciate that a rise in temperature may not be an early feature, and MHP should be considered in all cases of unexplained tachycardia, hyperventilation and sweating.

The aetiology of MHP lies in a complex intracellular abnormality of skeletal muscle metabolism. The central defect probably lies in the inability of the sarcoplasmic reticulum to take up calcium ions from the myoplasm. Mitochondrial function may also be defective with an inability to accumulate Ca^{2+} and there may also be an increased tendency for the muscle membrane to take up calcium ions from the extracellular fluid when the muscle membrane is exposed to a triggering agent.

In normal muscle physiology the actin and myosin filaments are prevented from being in a state of tonic contraction by the inhibitory action of troponin. When a contraction is initiated, calcium ions are released into the myoplasm where they combine with the troponin in such a way that the inhibitory effect of the troponin is removed. The actin and myosin can then form cross-filaments and thereby effect contraction.

When MHP is triggered the troponin is inactivated leading to continual muscle contracture and spasm. This vast increase in muscle metabolism results in muscle lactate production, heat production and a metabolic acidosis. The other resulting biochemical findings will be hyperkalaemia (acidosis and leakage from damaged muscle), hypocalcaemia (muscle uptake), reciprocal hypermagnesaemia and hyperphosphataemia (due to increased ATP breakdown in muscle).

In 90% of cases MHP is associated with the use of halothane or suxamethonium. Surgery should be discontinued and the patient ventilated with 100% oxygen using an Ambu bag and oxygen cylinder (i.e. removed from the halothane-contaminated machine). Rapid cooling should be instituted using cooled normal saline, ice packs for surface cooling and peritoneal dialysis with cooled dialysate solution. Large doses of sodium bicarbonate will be required to treat the acidosis, and the hyperkalaemia can be treated with a glucose and insulin infusion. Mannitol and frusemide are given to reduce the risk of renal tubular blockage from myoglobinuria. The definitive treatment is, however, dantrolene in a dose of 1–2 mg/kg up to a maximum of 10 mg/kg. The use of vasodilators such as glyceryl trinitrate or droperidol may be useful in promoting heat loss. The patient could be kept sedated and paralysed with the combination of an opiate and a non-depolarizing muscle relaxant which are not recognized triggering agents. Cardiac arrhythmias should be treated as appropriate, but calcium antagonist agents such as verapamil should be avoided.

The patient (and her family) should be investigated to confirm or refute the diagnosis. As there is no reliable screening test a muscle biopsy will need to be performed and the fresh muscle exposed to caffeine or halothane as triggering agents.

When this patient returns for further surgery, all recognized triggering agents should be avoided and a halothane-free machine used. The place of prophylactic dantrolene is controversial. Orally its absorption is poor and unreliable, and preoperatively an intravenous dose of 2.4 mg/kg is unpleasant; it may be just as reasonable to have the drug at hand while an appropriate technique is employed. Thiopentone and the opiates are 'safe', as too are the non-depolarizing muscle relaxants. However, neostigmine has been implicated so a short-acting agent such a atracurium that will not require reversal should be used. As hypercapnia per se has been shown to trigger the condition in pigs, spontaneous respiration should be avoided.

Although there was once a question mark over lignocaine, the Malignant Hyperthermia Association of the USA has declared the local analgesic drugs as safe. A spinal anaesthetic using bupivacaine would be ideal in this case. There are reports of dantrolene enhancing bupivacaine toxicity, but even if prophylaxis were given the small spinal dose would not render this a practical problem. Normal saline solution (not Hartmann's) should be used in preloading, and sympathomimetic agents such as ephedrine avoided if possible.

*A recent report from the CSM states that papaveretum should not be given to women of child-bearing potential.

Case 17

A 10-week-old baby was brought to the hospital. He had been vomiting increasingly over the past week, and over the previous 8 hours his mother felt that he had become increasingly pale and floppy. He had previously been well, following a normal delivery at term (weight 5.0 kg on admission).

On examination the baby was pale, cool and mottled peripherally. His pulse was 180 beats/min, regular, and the respiratory rate was 50/min. Blood test results showed a haemoglobin level of 9.9 g/dl, a white cell count of $6.2 \times 10^9/l$ and a platelet count of $212 \times 10^9/l$. Plasma electrolyte values were sodium 140 mmol/l, potassium 3.0 mmol/l, chloride 95 mmol/l, bicarbonate 32 mmol/l and urea 3.5 mmol/l.

Questions

1. Explain the biochemistry in terms of the most likely diagnosis.
2. How would you assess the degree of dehydration, and with what fluid would you resuscitate the baby?
3. If the extent of the circulatory collapse was so great that intravenous access could not be readily secured, do you know of any other route by which rapid volume repletion could be achieved?

4. Is the surgery urgent? How would you judge the best time to operate?

5. How would you induce anaesthesia? What size of endotracheal tube, which circuit, what flows and which ventilator would you use?

Discussion

The age of the baby, clinical presentation and the electrolyte findings make pyloric stenosis the most likely diagnosis. Persistent vomiting leads to the loss of gastric hydrochloric acid (HCl). This is produced by the action of carbonic anhydrase in the gastric mucosa with the reabsorption of bicarbonate (HCO_3^-) into the circulation. Thus as hydrogen ions are lost a metabolic alkalosis ensues. The concomitant reduction in the extracellular fluid leads to activation of the renin–angiotensin system and an increase in reabsorption by the proximal tubule in the kidney. However, due to the loss of chloride and the low level of chloride being presented to the proximal tubule, bicarbonate reabsorption is also increased under the action of carbonic anhydrase to permit maximal sodium retention. This leads to the paradox of an acidic urine being excreted in the presence of a metabolic alkalosis. The small amount of sodium remaining in the glomerular filtrate is then presented to the distal tubule operating under the influence of aldosterone, where sodium will be reabsorbed and potassium excreted. In severe fluid depletion the exchangeable pool of intracellular potassium will be depleted and under the influence of aldosterone the distal tubule will begin to excrete hydrogen ions in exhange for sodium, further worsening the alkalosis.

The degree of dehydration may be difficult to assess. Clues lie in the general condition and tone of the baby, the state of the mucous membranes, peripheral perfusion, core/peripheral temperature difference and the presence of a sunken anterior fontanelle. Another useful piece of information, if available, is a reliable, recent weight with which to compare the weight on admission.

Surgery is not urgent and should await rehydration and correction of the electrolyte abnormalities. The aim is to replace sodium, chloride and potassium. This will remove the renin and aldosterone influences from the kidney, whilst the repletion of chloride will allow the kidney to excrete bicarbonate. Prior to surgery it is necessary to correct the alkalaemia which if allowed to persist may cause postoperative apnoea. It has been demonstrated that the rise in the serum chloride level is a good indicator of the correction of the alkalaemia, and a target value for the chloride of 106 mmol/l has been suggested. Sodium, potassium and bicarbonate should then be in the normal range at the time of operation.

A haemoglobin value of 9–10 g/dl is appropriate at this stage, as the haemoglobin is reaching its physiological nadir with the transition from Hb-F to Hb-A, coupled with the reduced red cell survival of infancy. Initially the resuscitation fluid should be isotonic saline with the addition of potassium, later perhaps switching to half normal saline with glucose. Acetate-containing solutions should not be used as the acetate will be metabolized to bicarbonate in the liver and muscles; solutions of weak acid are almost never required.

As babies in such cases will be brought to theatre fully resuscitated with a gastric tube in place and an intravenous infusion in progress, it is probably best to aspirate the gastric tube and perform a rapid sequence induction, induce anaesthesia intravenously, intubate the baby with a 3.5 mm endotracheal tube and to ventilate, using a short-acting, non-depolarizing muscle relaxant with nitrous oxide and oxygen and a low concentration of volatile agent. An Ayre's T-piece should be used and the baby ventilated either by hand or using a ventilator such as the Nuffield Penlon fitted with a Newton valve which effectively converts it from a volume preset, time-cycled ventilator to a pressure-limited one. Fresh gas flow should be around 1000 ml plus 200 ml/kg to achieve normocapnia (assuming a ventilator frequency of around 20/min and a peak inflation pressure of around 20 cmH$_2$O). However, monitoring of the end-tidal carbon dioxide would be indicated. Opiates should be avoided if the baby is returning to a standard paediatric ward due to the increased sensitivity to respiratory depression. However, some thought should be given to postoperative analgesia: infiltration of the wound with bupivacaine is a useful manoeuvre.

In the event of severe circulatory collapse, in a child in whom it is proving impossible to establish satisfactory intravenous access, it is possible to give volume rapidly by the insertion of a needle intraosseously into the marrow, from which fluid will rapidly equilibrate with the intravascular volume. The generally favoured site for this is the upper tibia.

Case 18

A 21-year-old motor-cyclist was admitted to the accident and emergency department having been in collision with a car. He had sustained fractures of the left femur and pelvis. He also had extensive bruising over the left chest and a clinically obvious flail segment.

The patient was distressed and agitated. On examination he was found to be peripherally pale, shutdown, and centrally cyanosed. The pulse was regular, 135 beats/min, and the blood pressure was 110/90 mmHg. First and second heart sounds were normal; air entry to the left chest was reduced. The abdomen was soft; there was no focal neurology. The fractures were as described above.

The casualty officer relieved the agitation with 10 mg diazepam emulsion IV. However, the patient's colour deteriorated further; believing that extensive pulmonary contusion was present, the casualty officer gave suxamethonium, intubated the trachea and ventilated the patient.

The blood pressure disappeared.

Questions

1. What errors did the casualty officer make, and how would you retrieve the situation?
2. Following your intervention the patient returned to his previous state. What would you use for initial volume replacement?
3. How are colloids defined in physiochemical terms?
4. The patient's condition was stabilized, he was anaesthetized uneventfully for fixation of his fractures and ventilated overnight on the intensive care unit. The next morning he was awake and cooperative while being ventilated, warm and haemodynamic-ally stable. How would you manage him subsequently, bearing in mind his rib fractures?

Discussion

Hypoxia is frequently not appreciated as a cause of confusion and agitation in the traumatized patient, with the result that sedative agents may be given with disastrous consequences to hypoxic and hypovolaemic patients. This man might well have been hypoxic due to extensive pulmonary contusion, but the presence of rib fractures should have alerted the casualty officer to the possibility that a pneumothorax might be making a significant contribution to hypoxia. The rapid disappearance of the blood pressure with the commencement of artificial ventilation implies that a simple pneumothorax has been converted to a tension pneumothorax. The tension element is rapidly relieved by the insertion of a large-bore intravenous cannula into the second left intercostal space in the mid-clavicular line. This relieves the tension while preparations are made to insert a formal intercostal drain, to be connected to an underwater seal, for drainage of air and to re-expand the lung.

Simultaneous volume expansion should be in progress as these fractures and the associated chest injury could easily account for a 40% loss of the circulating blood volume, although the blood pressure may be maintained in a young, fit patient by intense vasoconstriction. In the UK most practitioners would probably commence resuscitation with a short-acting colloid solution of the gelatin group such as Haemacel or Gelofusine; the oncotically active molecules would initially confine the volume administered to the intravascular space. When a urea-linked gelatin such a Haemacel is used 30% of the molecules will be outside the circulation (extravascular) within 30 minutes, with the result that the volume-expanding half-life of the solution is relatively short, at around 2.5 hours. This is not necessarily a disadvantage, as later in the management it will be necessary to give blood to counteract the dilutional anaemia. If a colloid such as hetastarch with a long half-life (25 hours) had been used initially, the subsequent administration of blood could result in circulatory overload. In North America crystalloid fluids are favoured in the initial phase of resuscitation. However, as these will equilibrate freely with the interstitial and the intravascular space, they need to be given in a ratio of 3:1 to the volume of blood to be replaced. This will tend to result in a lowering of the colloid oncotic pressure (normal 25–30 mmHg) and may contribute to increased tissue oedema and possibly less effective gas exchange at the microcirculatory level.

Colloids may be defined in terms of their physiochemical properties, and these should be borne in mind in order to select the appropriate colloid for a particular clinical purpose. A colloid oncotic pressure is generated when a solution of colloid molecules is separated from its solvent by a semipermeable membrane, i.e. one that will impair the diffusion of colloid molecules across it but freely permit the movement of the solvent. Solvent is thus dragged towards the colloid side of the membrane. The magnitude of this colloid oncotic pressure (COP) is defined by the van't Hoff equation which states that the COP is proportional to the concentration of the colloid divided by the molecular weight. Thus the oncotic effect of a solution is proportional to the *number* of molecules in the solution, i.e. once the molecule is sufficiently large to prevent diffusion across the membrane, making it bigger does not increase the colloid oncotic effect but merely reduces the number of molecules that can be present at a given concentration. The maximum concentration possible in a clinical colloid solution will largely be governed by viscosity considerations. Thus the ideal colloid solution should have a narrow range of molecular sizes, just large enough to be retained by the capillary membrane.

In practice commercially prepared colloids contain a range of molecular sizes and are defined in terms of the oft-quoted but relatively meaningless 'weight average molecular weight', i.e. the mass of colloid divided by the number of molecules (typical values are 450 000 for hetastarch and 35 000 for the gelatins). At first sight this implies large, oncotically active molecules, but this average is skewed upwards by the presence of relatively few very large molecules. A more useful parameter is the 'number average molecular weight', which reflects the molecular weight of the most prevalent molecules within the solution (and remember it is the *number* of molecules that is important): values for hetastarch are 71 000 and for the gelatins 15 000. This value largely determines the propensity for a particular colloid to remain within the circulation, with the smaller molecules rapidly becoming extravascular or undergoing glomerular filtration. When gelatins are compared with albumin with a molecular weight of 69 000, it can be appreciated why the effect of the gelatins is relatively short-lived. Other factors, however, such as electrical charge do have a role and explain why, for instance, Gelofusine has a longer circulatory half-life than Haemaccel, despite having a similar range of molecular size. The use of larger molecular weight colloids such as hetastarch is more appropriate in situations of capillary leak where membrane permeabilities are increased. Their prolonged duration of action, however, makes the availability of the facility to measure colloid oncotic pressure increasingly important.

Commercially prepared colloids may also be compared in terms of the COPs they produce across commercially prepared membranes of different permeabilities – one permeable only to molecules of molecular weight less than 10 000 and the other permeable to molecules up to 50 000. This will generate COP_{10} and COP_{50} values. Thus solutions with a large number of relatively small molecules will have high COP_{10} but low COP_{50} values (e.g. Gelofusine), while those with fewer but larger molecules will have lower COP_{10} values but higher COP_{50} values. The ratio COP_{50}/COP_{10} is a reflection of the number of large molecules within a solution and reflects the tendency for it to remain intravascular (e.g. albumin 0.36, Haemaccel 0.18, hetastarch 0.58). This ratio is in effect analogous to (but not equivalent to) the Stavermann reflection coefficient, relating the hydrostatic and oncotic forces across the capillary membrane.

Fluid flux (Qf) across a semi-permeable capillary membrane is governed by the Starling equation:

$$Qf = Kf([Pmv\text{-}Ppmv] - \delta[\pi mv\text{-}\pi pmv])$$

where Kf is the filtration coefficient, Pmv and $Ppmv$ the microvascular and perimicrovascular pressures respectively and πmv and πpmv the colloid oncotic pressures of the microvascular and perimicrovascular spaces respectively. The Stavermann reflection coefficient (δ) is a measure of the permeability of that particular membrane for a particular molecule. When 1 the membrane is totally impermeable to the oncotically active molecule, when 0 completely permeable, e.g. the reflection coefficient of the pulmonary capillary endothelium for albumin is 0.6.

Early fixation of fractures may be important in reducing the incidence of fat emboli. The following morning this man appeared to be clinically ready to extubate; however, consideration must be given to the respiratory consequences of his fractured ribs and flail segment. In the past one approach has been to ventilate patients for a prolonged period to facilitate healing and prevent pulmonary collapse due to inability to cough and breathe deeply. Not only is this expensive and labour intensive, but it leaves the patient open to the risks of acquiring nosocomial infections such as pneumonia. Pulmonary collapse will, however, be prevented if the patient is provided with adequate analgesia to permit deep breathing and coughing. This would be a strong indication for thoracic epidural analgesia.

Case 19

A 35-year-old woman was found semicomatose with three empty tablet bottles at the bedside: these were labelled 'paracetamol', 'imipramine' and 'flunitrazepam'. She was last seen by her landlady 10 hours previously and appeared well.

On examination the woman was found to be warm and well perfused. The pulse was 60 beats/min, regular, with occasional dropped beats. The blood pressure was 100/60 mmHg, first and second heart sounds were normal and the chest was clear. The abdomen was soft. There were no focal neurological signs; the patient was making incomprehensible sounds, flexing and opening her eyes in response to painful stimuli, and gagging with pharyngeal wall stimulation. The ECG rhythm strip is shown in *Figure 19a*.

Questions

1. What is the nature of the ectopic beat on the rhythm strip?
2. How would you grade her level of consciousness?
3. Should the patient undergo gastric washout and if so, what precaution should be considered?
4. What antidotes are theoretically possible in this patient? Which would you give and which would you not give, and why?
5. What baseline investigations should be performed?
6. The patient is fully conscious 48 hours after admission but complains of abdominal pain and vomiting and is noted to be

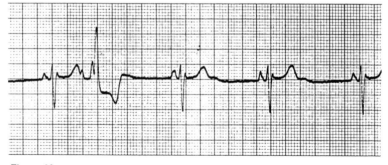

Figure 19a

jaundiced. Explain the mechanism of what has probably occurred and outline the subsequent management.

Discussion

The bizarre QRS complex is either a ventricular ectopic beat or an aberrantly conducted atrial ectopic beat. There are several clues to differentiating the two. Ventricular ectopic beats arise from ectopic foci in the ventricles and bear no relationship to preceding P waves. However, an aberrantly conducted atrial ectopic beat will be preceded by an abnormal atrial impulse or P' wave. Aberrantly conducted atrial ectopic beats arise when an atrial impulse meets a refractory right bundle but a recovered left bundle, and are thus transmitted through the ventricle with the characteristic RSR' pattern of right bundle branch block. They will also tend to occur early in the cycle following the previous sinus beat; i.e. early enough to find the right bundle still in its refractory period but not so early as to find both bundles refractory (in which case the result would be a non-conducted atrial ectopic beat). In contrast, a ventricular ectopic beat usually has a more bizarre configuration and the first upstroke is generally the tallest. This is sometimes known as the rule of 'rabbit ears': looking from behind, if the 'rabbit ear' on the left is taller than the 'rabbit ear' on the right then the likelihood is that it is a ventricular ectopic beat. The other possible clue to look for on the rhythm strip is to compare the distance between three normal sinus beats and the distance between two sinus beats interposed with an ectopic beat. With a ventricular ectopic beat the compensatory pause is complete, i.e. the interval between two sinus beats interposed by an ectopic beat will be equal to that between three sinus beats. If the ectopic beat is atrial in origin the distance will be less than that between three normal beats as the compensatory pause is incomplete.

Level of consciousness can be rapidly graded by use of the Glasgow coma scale: this allocates points on the basis of the best motor response, best verbal response and best ocular response (*Table 19a*). This patient would score 7.

We must assume that she has taken the overdose in the last 10 hours. Imipramine is a tricyclic antidepressant; this class of drugs possesses anticholinergic properties and will be likely to delay gastric emptying, making gastric lavage a worthwhile procedure.

It is a common mistake to assume that some evidence of a gag reflex ensures adequate airway protection in the unconscious

Table 19a   The Glasgow coma scale

	Score
Eye opening	
Spontaneously	4
Open to speech	3
Open to painful stimuli	2
Closed	1
Motor response	
Obeys commands	6
Localizes pain	5
Withdrawals to pain	4
Flexes to pain	3
Extends to pain	2
Nil	1
Verbal response	
Orientated	5
Confused	4
Inappropriate words	3
Incomprehensible sounds	2
Nil	1

patient. The protective laryngeal reflexes should not be regarded as an 'all or nothing' phenomenon; they will inevitably be significantly obtunded in a person with this degree of unconsciousness. Thus, in order to prevent the risk of pulmonary aspiration, she should be given a short-acting intravenous induction agent, suxamethonium, and intubated while cricoid pressure is applied. The endotracheal tube should remain in situ until there is no doubt regarding the patient's ability to protect her own airway.

Administering antidotes to all three of the agents involved in this overdose is theoretically possible but is not necessarily the appropriate treatment.

Paracetamol metabolism normally produces small amounts of a hepatotoxic metabolite, N-acetyl-p-benzoquinonimine. This is normally rapidly conjugated by glutathione. However, after an overdose glutathione stores will be depleted and excess metabolite can build up, leading to hepatic necrosis. The rate-limiting step for the synthesis of glutathione is the availability of cysteine. Thus administration of N-acetyl-cysteine will allow the regeneration of glutathione, and if given up to 8–10 hours following the overdose should prevent hepatic necrosis. Starting the infusion need not await a paracetamol level; it should be continued if the level is above the toxicity threshold with respect to time (*Figure 19b*).

The anticholinergic side-effects of the tricyclic antidepressants may result in cardiac arrhythmias in overdosage and these could theoretically be dealt with using an anticholinergic agent such as physostigmine. However, because of all the other problems associated with physostigmine such as excess salivation, bradycardia and bronchoconstriction, its use should be reserved for the life-threatening situation when conventional antiarrhythmic drugs have failed.

Flumazenil has recently been developed to antagonize the sedative effect of the benzodiazepines at the gamma amino butyric acid (GABA) receptor. However, benzodiazepines are very safe even in overdose and supportive treatment is all that is generally required. In addition flumazenil is a short-acting drug compared with its agonists, and in the overdose setting would have to be given by continuous infusion, entailing considerable expense. A further danger of benzodiazepine reversal in this case is that it may unmask the epileptogenic effect of the tricyclic antidepressant and result in fitting.

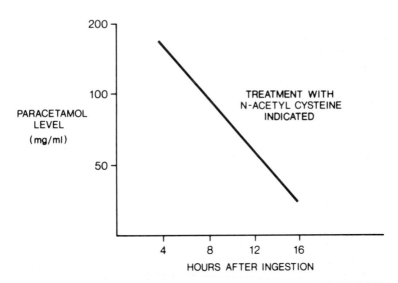

Figure 19b Indication for acetylcysteine treatment in paracetamol overdose

In addition to a paracetamol level, baseline levels of liver function tests and clotting indices should be obtained in view of the possibility of delayed hepatic necrosis.

After 48 hours the patient appears to be developing acute hepatic necrosis, despite treatment with acetylcysteine. It is entirely possible that the paracetamol was taken the day before the overdose of sedative agents. Paracetamol overdose accounts for 50% of acute liver failure in the UK; it carries a poor prognosis, and early referral to a liver unit is recommended. The disease progression is best monitored by serial prothrombin times, as the clotting factors have shorter half-lives than the serum albumin. Liver enzyme levels are of little value; high levels are suggestive of severe damage, but low levels may represent a severely damaged, 'burnt-out' liver. Encephalopathy may develop rapidly but its mechanism is obscure. Failure of deamination leads to azotaemia and the build-up of other compounds which in some way interfere with neuronal energy metabolism or disrupt the blood–brain barrier, rendering it permeable to other toxins. Encephalopathy is aggravated by the absorption of nitrogen from the gut; protein should therefore be excluded from the diet, purging instituted with lactulose, and H_2-receptor antagonists given to try to reduce gastrointestinal haemorrhage.

Episodic cerebral oedema may complicate grade IV encephalopathy. Renal failure complicates 75% of cases and early haemodialysis may improve the prognosis. It is aimed to keep the plasma osmolality below 320 mosmol/kg. H_2O. Ventilatory support may be needed, and pulmonary oedema is particularly likely in paracetamol overdose cases complicated by metabolic acidosis. The circulatory picture is akin to that of septic shock with a high cardiac output but a low systemic vascular resistance.

It must be stressed, however, that the management of these very sick patients should be undertaken in a dedicated liver unit and early consideration given to liver transplantation.

Case 20

A 53-year-old woman with osteoarthritis of the hip required a total hip replacement. The past history revealed that she had been unwell in her teens, when she was treated with 3 months' bed rest. Over the past 10 years she had become increasingly short of breath with exertion, although she did not complain of any anginal symptoms.

Cardiovascular examination revealed an irregular pulse of 90 beats/min, blood pressure of 105/85 mmHg, and first and second heart sounds. In addition, the houseman thought that he could hear either a third heart sound or a diastolic murmur. Fine, bilateral basal crepitations were noted. The patient's medication consisted of Digoxin 0.25 mg, bendrofluazide 5 mg and warfarin 3 mg once daily, and cimetidine 200 mg and ibuprofen 400 mg three times daily. The following test results were obtained:

Full blood count: haemoglobin 12.0 g/dl, white cell count $5.9 \times 10^9/l$, platelets $230 \times 10^9/l$
Urea and electrolytes: sodium 129 mmol/l, potassium, 2.8 mmol/l, bicarbonate 30 mmol/l, urea 8.2 mmol/l
Glucose 11.2 mmol/l
Prothrombin time 54 s (control 12 s)

The ECG rhythm strip is shown in *Figure 20a*, and the chest X-ray in *Figure 20b*.

Questions

1. What cardiac lesion does this woman suffer from? Did the houseman hear a third heart sound or a diastolic murmur? Explain the mechanism of the dyspnoea in pathophysiological terms.
2. Can you explain the biochemistry? Should the low sodium concentration be treated? What potential problems might the low potassium level cause?
3. Why might this patient be hyperglycaemic?
4. Suggest a reason for the excessive anticoagulation.

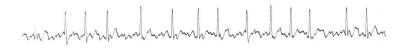

Figure 20a

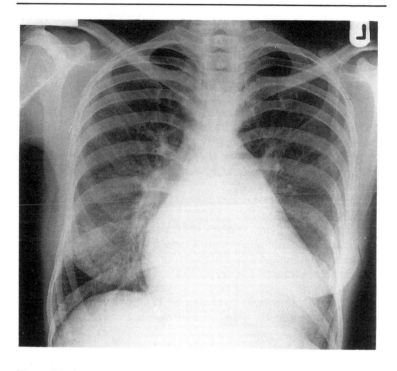

Figure 20b

5. Do you think that spinal anaesthesia would be suitable in this patient?
6. What particular considerations would govern your conduct of a general anaesthetic?
7. Would you use a flow-directed pulmonary artery catheter?

Discussion

This patient has mitral stenosis. The history is strongly suggestive of an episode of rheumatic fever. As the left atrial pressure rises behind the stenotic mitral valve, fluid is progressively dammed back leading to a chronic rise in the pulmonary venous pressure and the development of interstitial oedema. This reduces the pulmonary compliance and leads to the sensation of dyspnoea. Finally, when the rate of fluid formation exceeds the drainage capacity of the pulmonary lymphatics, frank intra-alveolar pulmonary oedema develops. The chest X-ray supports the diagnosis, with evidence of left atrial enlargement in the presence of pulmonary venous congestion. Kerley's lines above the costophrenic angles should be looked for, but are difficult to visualize in this radiograph (*Figure 20b*).

The houseman must have heard a diastolic murmur; a third heart sound (due to atrial contraction) is impossible in atrial fibrillation as there is no atrial contraction. Remember that the severity of the lesion is proportional to the *length* of the murmur and the presence of an early opening snap, rather than to the loudness of the murmur.

The electrolyte levels suggest that this woman is chronically hypokalaemic with a compensatory metabolic alkalosis. This has probably resulted from treatment with thiazide diuretic drugs. The thiazide is probably also responsible for the elevated glucose level. Digoxin toxicity is exhanced in the presence of hypokalaemia and there may well be impaired renal clearance of the drug. It would be meddlesome, and wrong, to attempt to treat the low sodium which has fallen appropriately in an attempt to maintain a normal plasma osmolality in the face of a rise in the glucose and urea concentrations.

Anticoagulant therapy should aim at producing a prolongation of the prothrombin time of between two and three times the control value. This patient is grossly over-anticoagulated, probably as a result of warfarin metabolism being retarded owing to inhibition of the hepatic P450 enzyme system by cimetidine.

Two reasons make spinal anaesthesia inappropriate in this case. Firstly, anticoagulant therapy predisposes to the risk of epidural haematoma formation. Secondly, spinal anaesthesia may result in sudden and uncontrollable vasodilatation leading to systemic hypotension. The heart in mitral stenosis will be unable to compensate for this by an increase in the cardiac output.

Severe mitral stenosis is effectively a fixed cardiac output state with a very limited ability to compensate for changes in 'afterload' and 'preload'. Similarly, extremes of tachycardia and bradycardia are poorly tolerated. Therefore the cornerstone of a good anaesthetic technique is the maintenance of cardiovascular stability. Heart rate should be maintained as near to normal as possible and there should be meticulous fluid replacement (under central venous pressure control) to maintain the right atrial pressure. Solutions of vasoconstrictors such as phenylephrine should be immediately to hand to treat episodes of systemic hypotension.

This is not, however, an indication for light anaesthesia, as exaggerated sympathoadrenal responses to surgical stimulation would be equally deleterious.

The role of the pulmonary artery catheter is debatable. It will provide useful measurements of cardiac output and systemic vascular resistance, and permit the rational use of inotropes and vasoconstrictors on the basis of haemodynamic variables. However, in the presence of a stenotic mitral valve, pulmonary artery occlusion pressure readings may be a poor reflection of the filling pressure of the left side of the heart, and the risk of pulmonary haemorrhage should be seriously considered in a patient with pulmonary hypertension receiving anticoagulants.

Case 21

A 60-year-old woman with an unremarkable medical history, including one previous uneventful anaesthetic for a cholecystectomy, was anaesthetized for a total hip replacement. She was starved preoperatively and given diazepam 10 mg as a premedicant. Anaesthesia was induced (fentanyl 150 μg, thiopentone 300 mg, alcuronium 20 mg), and a cuffed endotracheal tube was passed with ease. She was transferred to the operating theatre and connected to a Manley ventilator delivering nitrous oxide and oxygen plus halothane at a fresh gas flow of 6 litres per minute. The pulse oximeter indicated a saturation of 99%. She was turned on her side and the operation commenced. Shortly afterwards the ventilator started to 'judder' and the weight failed to 'bottom out'. The saturation fell to 88% and on listening to the chest wheezing was noted.

Questions

1. What are the possible causes? What sequence of events should you go through to establish the cause and rectify the situation?
2. Can aspiration pneumonitis be ruled out in this situation?
3. What is the likelihood of this being an allergic reaction to an anaesthetic agent? What types of 'allergic' reaction do you recognize?

4. Outline the management of a suspected hypersensitivity reaction.

Discussion

The important point to appreciate here is that this patient has not necessarily developed true bronchospasm within the small airways, and that reaching for the aminophylline is not the appropriate reflex response.

The fact that the problem has arisen immediately following the change of the position from supine to lateral should alert the anaesthetist to the possibility of a problem relating to the position of the endotracheal tube. It may have become kinked during the turn: is it possible to pass a suction catheter? Its position may have been advanced resulting in an endobronchial intubation, which interestingly often causes bronchospasm. Another possibility always to be borne in mind is cuff herniation; this will readily be cured by deflating the cuff. If, after taking over ventilation manually, the patient still proves impossible to ventilate, the tube should be removed and the patient ventilated by bag and mask: *if in doubt, take it out.*

Careful auscultation of the chest should diagnose an endobronchial intubation. If a marked discrepancy between right and left-sided air entry persists after pulling back the tube to a point where it is definitely within the trachea, serious consideration should be given to the possibility of a pneumothorax. If this is thought likely, nitrous oxide should be discontinued (as it will tend to increase the volume of the pneumothorax due to its greater diffusibility).

In practice it takes a very short time to go through a drill to eliminate these possible causes. At this point it would be reasonable to assume that the bronchospasm has its aetiology in the smaller airway. Deepening the anaesthesia with halothane may be all that is required, whilst aminophylline is still arguably the best first-line agent for specific management.

Aspiration pneumonitis can never be wholly ruled out as a cause of bronchospasm. Aspiration pneumonitis classically produces wheeze and cyanosis rather than crepitations. Starving elective patients for 4–6 hours preoperatively increases the likelihood of an empty stomach, but there is no patient in whom an empty stomach can be guaranteed as the rate of gastric emptying shows very marked interindividual variation. Hiatus hernia is often undiagnosed. Rules for starvation periods are welded into tradition but have little foundation in physiology; they are, incidentally, often unnecessarily prolonged in small children and babies. Similarly the presence of a cuffed endotracheal tube is no guarantee that the airway will be protected from soiling. The high-volume, low-pressure cuffs used to prevent excessive tracheal wall pressure are notorious in this respect, and have been shown to permit the passage of dye along the folds in the cuff material. Foam cuffed endotracheal tubes may be preferable in this respect.

Hypersensitivity to an intravenous anaesthetic agent is unlikely to be the aetiology in this case, although the possibility of idiosyncratic reactions should be borne in mind with the administration of any anaesthetic agent.

'Allergy' is probably the most misused word in the medical dictionary, and the classification and nomenclature relating to so-called allergic reactions to anaesthetic agents is potentially one of the most confusing areas of anaesthetic practice. Idiosyncratic reactions to agents may initially be divided into two groups. Firstly, and more straightforwardly, there is the exaggerated pharmacological response; for example, 250 mg thiopentone will cause a modest fall in blood pressure when given to a fit patient, but the same dose given to an elderly hypovolaemic patient, will probably result in a catastrophic fall in blood pressure. However, this is merely relative overdosage and should not occur if there is full appreciation of the circumstances of the case. There will be no other features such as urticaria, bronchospasm or laryngeal oedema to suggest ongoing immunological activation. This should not really be classed as an adverse reaction to thiopentone and certainly not as an allergic one.

Hypersensitivity reactions when immunological mechanisms are brought into play may be termed 'anaphylactic' or 'anaphylactoid'. Strictly speaking, the term 'anaphylactic' should be confined to an immunologically mediated type I hypersensitivity reaction where antibodies of the IgE class (bound to the surface of mast cells) are sensitized to an intravenous agent. Subsequent exposure to the agent results in the drug binding to the IgE on the surface of the mast cell, causing mast cell degranulation and the release of histamine along with other cytotoxic mediators. This will result in the classical features of acute anaphylaxis: profound hypotension (the associated vasodilatation and capillary leak may result in the rapid loss of 2 litres from the circulating volume), bronchospasm and urticarial rash.

Other hypersensitivity reactions may be brought about by different immunological mechanisms. These may involve complement activation via the classical pathway following sensitization with other classes of immunoglobulin such as IgG. Complement may also be activated directly at the C3a point (the so-called alternate pathway) leading to histamine release, while many drugs have the capacity to cause the direct release of histamine. These latter reactions will be clinically indistinguishable from acute anaphylaxis and are termed 'anaphylactoid'. The term 'anaphylaxis' should be reserved for reactions proved to be due to type I immediate hypersensitivity involving mast cell-bound IgE, which almost be definition implies previous exposure to the drug. Anaphylactoid reactions may occur without previous exposure to the drug and may equally well occur after several uneventful exposures.

Hypersensitivity reactions are rare, with an overall incidence of 1 in 5000 to 1 in 20 000. In this respect alcuronium is perhaps the most frequently implicated non-depolarizing muscle relaxant. The vast majority of such reactions tend to occur within 5 minutes of injecting the offending agent, and the most frequent feature is cardiovascular collapse with a rash. Nevertheless, delayed onset is recognized and isolated bronchospasm may occasionally be the only feature. The first-line treatment of acute anaphylactic or anaphylactoid reactions involves the rapid administration of colloid and the early use of the physiological antagonist of histamine, namely adrenaline. The use of the pharmacological antagonist (i.e. an antihistamine) will be of little benefit, as the histamine will have bound to its receptors; the only value of an antihistamine would be to block those receptors not bound with histamine or to prevent subsequent binding.

Subsequent attention is directed towards establishing the precise cause of the reaction. Serial blood samples should be collected into EDTA tubes for assays of IgE and complement levels, which in association with white cell counts and differentials may elucidate the precise mechanism. Patch testing may implicate the offending agent.

Case 22

A 70-year-old man was found to have an operable carcinoma of the rectum. Over the past 10 years, however, he had become progressively short of breath and was only able to walk some 50–100 metres on the flat before he had to stop to recover his breath. The previous year he was admitted to hospital with a further exacerbation of his dyspnoea, at which time he was found to have a pneumothorax which responded to treatment with a chest drain connected to an underwater seal. His medication consisted of sustained-release aminophylline 225 mg twice daily, and cimetidine 400 mg at night (empirically for dyspepsia).

On examination the patient had a regular pulse of 100 beats/min, and blood pressure of 130/80 mmHg. First and second heart sounds were barely audible. Other findings were mild dyspnoea at rest, pursed lips breathing; chest movement was poor, percussion note bilaterally hyperresonant and a fine expiratory wheeze was audible throughout both lung fields. Laboratory investigations gave the following values:

Full blood count: haemoglobin 13.5 g/dl, white cell count 7.5×10^9/l, platelet count 50×10^9/l
Urea and electrolytes were normal
Arterial blood gases (taken breathing air): pH 7.38, P_{O_2} 9.2 kPa, P_{CO_2} 4.8 kPa, standard bicarbonate 28 mmol/l, base excess 0 mmol/l

The chest X-ray is shown in *Figure 22a*, and the pulmonary function tests in *Table 22a*

Questions

1. Suggest a cause, and a possible remedy, for the thrombocytopenia.
2. How would you characterize the respiratory defect demonstrated by the spirometry?
3. What technique may have been used to determine the ratio of residual volume (RV) to the total lung capacity (TLC)? Comment on the significance of the result.
4. What further piece of information, measurable at the bedside, would make the interpretation of the blood gases more meaningful?
5. Do you think there is potential for improvement preoperatively?
6. What major intraoperative problem should be anticipated, and what monitoring would you employ?

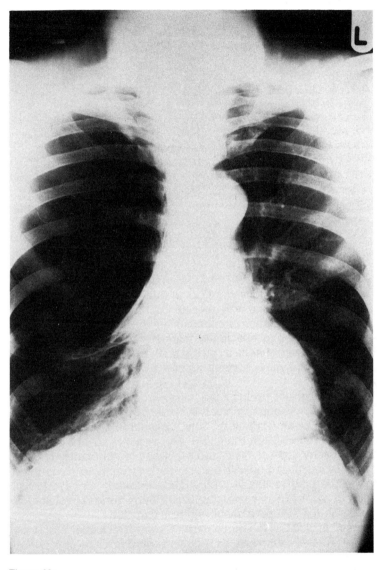

Figure 22a

Table 22a   Results of pulmonary function tests

	Control	Post salbutamol
PEFR (l/min)	60	98
FEV$_1$/FVC (l)	0.8/2.0	1.1/2.1
RV/TLC (l)	5.5/8.0	N/A
CO transfer factor (ml/min/mmHg) normal 20–38 ml/min/mmHg	5	

PEFR, peak expiratory flow rate; FEV$_1$, forced expiratory flow rate in 1 second; FVC, forced vital capacity; RV, residual volume; TLC, total lung capacity; CO, carbon monoxide.

7. Identify the major postoperative consideration, and outline your approach.

Discussion

The thrombocytopenia may well be a side-effect of the cimetidine, and since the patient was placed on this empirically without endoscopic confirmation of peptic ulceration it should probably be stopped in order to see if the platelet count recovers spontaneously. Another potential problem that the cimetidine might cause is theophylline toxicity as the result of hepatic enzyme inhibition.

This man's major problem is severe chronic obstructive airways disease. The spirometry reveals a marked obstructive defect with a very low peak expiratory flow rate, a reduced FEV$_1$ and a FEV$_1$/FVC ratio of less than 75%. The residual volume and total lung capacity are not measurable by simple spirometry but are generally calculated using a helium dilution technique. Hyperinflation of the lung results in a high TLC, and early airway closure leads to extensive gas trapping and a large residual volume. In health the RV/TLC ratio should be less than 40%.

Taken in isolation the blood gases are unremarkable. This is the picture of severe emphysema: a patient who lies at the 'pink puffer' end of the spectrum of chronic obstructive airways disease. In pathophysiological terms this is the disease of massive dead space. What would be useful to know, however, is what order of minute volume (and hence some indication of the work of breathing) the patient is required to generate in order to achieve sufficient alveolar ventilation in the face of a massive dead space to maintain acceptable oxygenation and normocapnia. This could be measured simply at the bedside using a tightly fitting mask connected to a Wright's spirometer.

Frequently the airways obstruction in emphysema is fixed, offering little opportunity for useful pharmacological intervention. There is no evidence of infection and so antibiotics are not indicated. However, there is evidence of a bronchodilator response to salbutamol. It would be worthwhile to attempt to optimize bronchodilator therapy preoperatively using both sympathomimetic and anticholinergic agents, and possibly consider a trial of steroids.

The chest X-ray (*Figure 22a*) shows the hyperexpanded, lucent lungs of emphysema. There is also a large emphysematous bulla occupying the majority of the right lung field. The history of this man's previous admission suggests that the bulla had ruptured on that occasion. Thus mechanical ventilation may well result in a further episode of rupture and the development of a preoperative pneumothorax, for which a high index of suspicion should be maintained throughout the procedure. In view of this, and the underlying pathology, the patient requires a ventilator that will deliver a sufficient minute volume to achieve adequate gas exchange with the lowest possible inflation pressures. Adequate time needs to be allowed for full expiration and the facility to vary the inspiratory:expiratory ratio could be useful. A high-frequency jet ventilator such as the Bromsgrove ventilator might fit the bill, but effective gas exchange would be difficult to measure and frequent blood gas sampling would be necessary to ensure normocapnia. Even with a more conventional ventilator, capnography will have its limitations as there will be an increased alveolar to arterial gradient for carbon dioxide and an arterial line for blood gas analysis would be indicated in any case. A high index of suspicion for pneumothorax should be maintained throughout the procedure.

The major consideration postoperatively is the fact that pain and sedation may well render the patient unable to achieve his normally high minute volume, which is obligatory to maintain adequate gas exchange. In general terms postoperative ventilation should be avoided in this group of patients, but a short period may be required particularly after major abdominal or thoracic procedures if adequate spontaneous ventilation cannot be established. This would ideally be a gradual weaning process from a machine offering a sophisticated weaning mode such as synchronized intermittent mandatory ventilation (SIMV) with pressure support. This will allow the patient gradually to increase his own contribution to the minute volume as sedative drugs wear off and effective analgesia is established. Thoracic epidural analgesia would be strongly indicated, but would be precluded if the thrombocytopenia had not responded to the withdrawal of cimetidine. Consideration should also be given to the nutritional needs of the patient to prevent wasting of the respiratory muscles. The enteral route is by far the most preferable, but if prolonged ileus looks like making this option unavailable, then consideration should be given to early intravenous feeding. With respect to feeding regimens, it may be useful to increase the proportion of energy given as fat as opposed to carbohydrate; the complete oxygenation of fat results in less carbon dioxide production than does the metabolism of carbohydrate. This may be important in patients whose ability to eliminate carbon dioxide is critical. The respiratory quotient (the ratio of carbon dioxide production to oxygen consumption) may vary from 0.7 on a total fat diet to 1.0 on a diet consisting solely of carbohydrate.

Case 23

The man shown in the photograph (*Figure 23a*) presented to his general practitioner complaining of headache and visual disturbance. He required corrective surgery for the condition.

On examination a regular pulse of 70 beats/min and blood pressure of 180/110 mmHg were noted. First and second heart sounds were normal. The chest was clinically clear. A full blood count was normal. Other values were: sodium 138 mmol/l, potassium 4.4 mmol/l, chloride 100 mmol/l, bicarbonate 24 mmol/l, urea 5.2 mmol/l and glucose 11.4 mmol/l. The ECG is shown in *Figure 23b* and the nuclear magnetic resonance scan in *Figure 23c*.

Questions

1. What is this man's condition? What do the nuclear magnetic resonance scan and the ECG show?

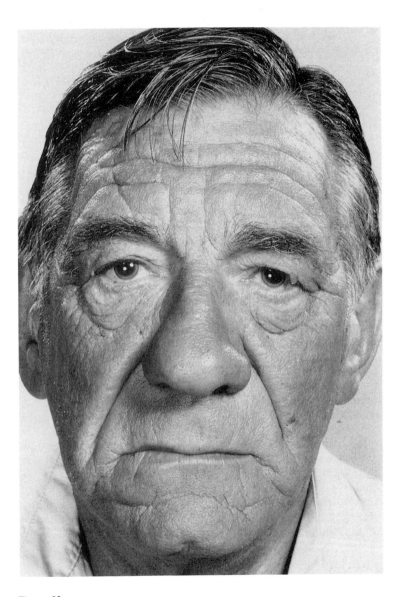

Figure 23a

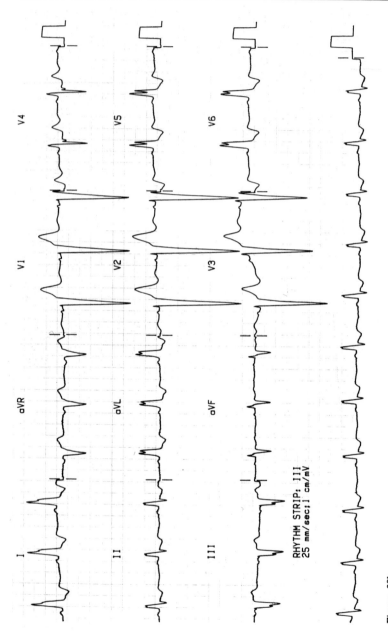

Figure 23b

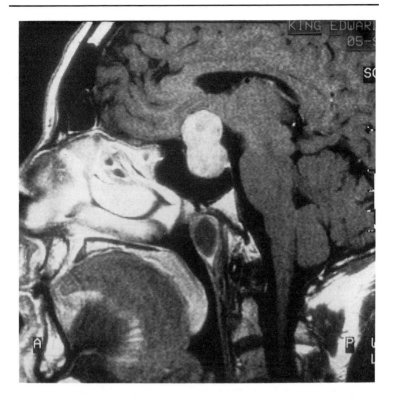

Figure 23c

2. Explain and suggest a cause for the metabolic abnormality.
3. What other investigations might you require preoperatively?
4. What anaesthetic problems should be anticipated?
5. How should the postoperative period be managed?
6. The following electrolyte levels are reported postoperatively: sodium 155 mmol/l, potassium 4.3 mmol/l, bicarbonate 28 mmol/l, urea 9.6 mmol/l. Plasma osmolality is 330 /mosmol/kg/H_2O. What do you suspect, and how would you confirm it?

Discussion

The nuclear magnetic resonance (NMR) scan shows a pituitary adenoma which coupled with the clinical appearance suggests a diagnosis of acromegaly. This is due to the overproduction of growth hormone by an adenoma in the anterior pituitary. As growth hormone is a catabolic hormone and has anti-insulin actions a significant proportion of these patients have impaired glucose tolerance or frank diabetes. Although the anaesthetist should be aware of this, the level of hyperglycaemia in this patient should not cause any particular problems.

However, there are a number of other important considerations that the anaesthetist needs to be aware of. These patients are frequently hypertensive and are also subject to a progressive cardiomyopathy. In this instance the ECG shows left bundle branch block which makes other electrocardiographic diagnoses such as left ventricular hypertrophy difficult, or even impossible. Lung volumes are large and there is alteration in the V/Q relationships within the lung. Despite initial muscle hypertrophy this can progress to a myopathy and postoperative respiratory problems should be anticipated.

The most important considerations, however, probably relate to the management of the airway. There is extensive overgrowth of pharyngeal and laryngeal structures and a number of patients may be frankly stridulous. Airway maintenance and intubation may be extremely difficult and necessitate consideration being given to awake fibreoptic intubation or even the performance of a tracheostomy under local anaesthesia.

It is relatively unusual for pituitary adenomas to result in mass effects such as the obstruction of cerebrospinal fluid flow and the development of raised intracranial pressure, but the possibility should be borne in mind. More relevant, however, is the effect of an expanding pituitary adenoma on the production of other pituitary hormones: most importantly, there could be reduced adrenocorticotrophic hormone (ACTH) production and impairment of the stress response to surgery and anaesthesia. Similarly, thyroid stimulating hormone (TSH) production could be impaired, leading to secondary myxoedema which classically may result in extreme sensitivity to sedative agents generally. A case could be made for a preoperative thyroxine estimation and an assessment of the adrenocortical–pituitary axis; this would generally take the form of an insulin stress test and measurement of the cortisol response to hypoglycaemia. However, these patients will be treated with steroid cover before and after surgery, and such specific tests are of somewhat academic value (and not without their changes).

The NMR scan shows a large adenoma with suprasellar extension. Older teaching was that such extensive lesions would require a frontal craniotomy to achieve their removal. However, such lesions are now increasingly being removed via the transsphenoidal approach. Considerable bleeding should be anticipated with this technique.

Postoperatively, hormone replacement should be continued with glucocorticoids and possibly thyroxine. Mineralocorticoids should theoretically not be needed as the aldosterone-producing area of the adrenal cortex, the zona glomerulosa, is under the influence of the renin–angiotensin system.

Diabetes insipidus is another potential postoperative complication that should be anticipated, and is suggested by the postoperative electrolyte values if they occur in the setting of a high urine output. Antidiuretic hormone (ADH) from the posterior pituitary is released in response to a rising plasma osmolality and acts on the distal tubule of the kidney rendering it permeable to water. Failure of ADH is confirmed when the plasma osmolality is inappropriately high in the presence of a dilute urine of low osmolality. There should then be a dramatic response to the administration of a synthetic analogue such as desmopressin (DDAVP).

Case 24

A 19-year-old primigravida had been in hospital for 2 weeks. Over the preceding 24 hours her blood pressure had risen from 150/100 mmHg to 190/120 mmHg. She had become 'twitchy', mildly photophobic and grossly oedematous. The obstetricians wished to deliver her expeditiously by Caesarean section under general anaesthesia. The urine output was noted to have declined.

Blood test results were sodium 130 mmol/l, potassium 4.2 mmol/l, bicarbonate 25 mmol/l and urea 6.9 mmol/l.

Questions

1. What is the diagnosis?
2. How could you gain a better indication of this patient's renal function?
3. How and why do both the physiological changes of pregnancy and her disease state cause you to modify your general anaesthetic technique compared with the non-pregnant state?

Discussion

This woman has pre-eclamptic toxaemia (PET): a triad of oedema, proteinuria (more than 300 mg per day) and hypertension arising after the 28th week of gestation. Severe cases may progress to the rapid development of cerebral oedema and eclamptic fitting. The increased extracellular volume and the systemic hypertension may precipitate cardiac failure, whilst the glomerular damage indicated by the proteinuria may progress to acute renal failure. A rapidly developing coagulopathy may also be a feature which, if present, will preclude the use of epidural anaesthesia and analgesia in these patients. The precise aetiology remains unclear but may in part lie in an inappropriate immunological response to placental tissues.

Recent work suggests that low-dose aspirin may have a therapeutic role in PET by suppressing the production of thromboxane A_2 (a potent vasoconstrictor). Aspirin may, however, increase the bleeding tendency, and the approach to the patient on low-dose aspirin requesting epidural anaesthesia will pose the obstetric anaesthetist a new problem if this treatment comes into widespread use.

This patient's renal function should give cause for concern. Although her serum urea level is only at the upper end of the normal range it may be regarded as elevated in a pregnant patient when the urea will normally tend to fall as a result both of the increased glomerular filtration rate and dilution due to the expansion of the extracellular space. Measuring and calculating the creatinine clearance will give a better idea of the renal function. This will however require a 24-hour urine collection and a measurement of the serum creatinine. The following formula is then applied:

$$C_{cp} = \frac{(U_{cr}) \times V}{(P_{cr}) \times t}$$

where C_{cp} is the creatinine clearance in ml/min, U_{cr} is the concentration of creatinine in the urine, P_{cr} is the concentration of creatinine in the plasma, V is the volume of urine and t is the period of the collection.

Creatinine is produced at a fairly constant rate in proportion to the muscle mass. It is not reabsorbed by the renal tubules and there is little tubular secretion. Thus the creatinine clearance can be approximated to the glomerular filtration rate.

We could also look at the sodium content of the urine. An absent or low concentration of urinary sodium would indicate that the renal tubules still have the ability to retain sodium. These results would be negated by any prior administration of loop diuretics such as frusemide.

Essentially three considerations cause us to modify our general anaesthetic technique for Caesarean section in this patient compared with (say) anaesthesia for a cholecystectomy in the same patient:

1. The physiological changes of pregnancy.
2. Further pathophysiological considerations as a result of pre-eclampsia.
3. Fetal considerations.

From the early stages of pregnancy all pregnant patients are at risk of regurgitation and the subsequent aspiration of gastric contents. There is a reduction in the tone of the lower oesophageal sphincter mediated by the smooth muscle relaxant effects of progesterone. This patient will require a rapid sequence induction and the application of cricoid pressure. Preoperatively efforts should be made to reduce gastric acidity to a pH of 2.5 or greater; prior to an emergency Caesarean section, this will involve the administration of an H_2-receptor antagonist such as ranitidine to block the further production of acid. This will take about 20 minutes to be effective following intravenous administration. However, it will have no neutralizing effect on acid already within the stomach, and a single dose of a non-particulate antacid such as sodium citrate should be administered for this purpose. These agents are now preferred to particulate antacids such as magnesium trisilicate, as it has been suggested that inhalation of particulate matter may produce a pneumonitis in its own right.

There is an increase in tidal volume and a reduction in the functional residual capacity in pregnancy which results in a reduction in the nitrogen wash-out time and implies that the time necessary for preoxygenation may be reduced to around 3 minutes. However, the downside of this change is that the oxygen stores of the mother are reduced at a time of increased metabolic demand. Thus in the setting of a failed intubation cyanosis will appear earlier at a time when the duration of suxamethonium may well be prolonged owing to the relative lack of pseudocholine-sterase in pregnancy.

Sedative premedication is to be avoided because of the risks of fetal accumulation. Albumin-bound drugs such as diazepam will tend to accumulate in the fetus and result in fetomaternal ratios in excess of unity. Being lipid-soluble, all intravenous induction agents will cross the placenta and there is probably little to choose between them in this respect. In general, opiates are avoided prior to the delivery of the baby. For many years it has been traditional to administer an inspired oxygen concentration of at least 50% prior to delivery in the belief that the Apgar scores of the baby would be better. However, there is no evidence, on the basis of umbilical artery pH values, that this practice offers any advantage over 30% oxygen. Using 30% oxygen permits the use of 70% nitrous oxide and thus tends to reduce the hazard of awareness. In a similar vein it was traditional to avoid volatile agents during Caesarean section and instead to 'anaesthetize' using hyperventilation to low levels of $P\text{CO}_2$ using nitrous oxide and oxygen. These techniques led to caesarean section being associated with high levels of awareness, which has attracted much adverse publicity in recent years. Routine anaesthesia for a Caesarean section should now involve the administration of a volatile supplement to eliminate the possibility of awareness. The previous considerations were probably erroneous anyway in terms of fetal protection, as 'light' anaesthesia will precipitate an outpouring of catecholamines which will result in vasoconstriction within the uteroplacental bed. Modest hyperventilation is employed to maintain the physiological lowering of the $P\text{CO}_2$ which provides the diffusion gradient down which the fetus can eliminate carbon dioxide. It should always be remembered that a lateral tilt is maintained throughout prior to delivery, thus avoiding aortocaval compression.

In this patient the presence of moderately severe PET imposes some further considerations on the technique of anaesthesia. The presence of peripheral oedema may prevent an appreciation of the fact that there is depletion of the intravascular space and relative hypovolaemia. The Starling forces across the capillary membrane are disrupted and the low serum albumin results in a lowering of the colloid oncotic pressure. This, coupled with the increased cardiovascular demands of pregnancy, places these patients at great risk of acute pulmonary oedema. Consideration should be given to controlled volume expansion, preferably with a long-acting colloid solution (arguably salt-poor 20% albumin solution to increase the oncotic pressure and to mobilize oedema fluid from the interstitial to the intravascular space). Consideration could be given to the use of 'renal' doses of dopamine in an endeavour to preserve renal function. If renal function is thought to be impaired then atracurium would be the non-depolarizing muscle relaxant of choice and arguably enflurane should be avoided. Enflurane metabolism will produce free fluoride ions up to a concentration of 20 μmol/l after 2–3 hours of anaesthesia. However, this is still below the threshold for renal tubular toxicity which is thought to lie around 50 μmol/l (cf. methoxyflurane).

The greatest cause of maternal mortality in association with pre-eclampsia is an intracerebral catastrophe as a result of failure to control the blood pressure. Obstetricians have traditionally used hydralazine for this purpose, but reflex tachycardia may be a problem. Other agents such as labetalol and nifedipine may have a useful role either alone or in combination.

From the strictly anaesthetic point of view the greatest risk lies in precipitating a dangerous hypertensive response at laryngoscopy and intubation. There are a number of possible agents that may be used to try to attenuate this response, such as labetalol or lignocaine, but none is wholly reliable. The most reliable approach would seem to be the use of a potent intravenous opiate, and there is probably little to choose between fentanyl and alfentanil here. The price will be respiratory depression in the neonate, but this can be readily dealt with by the paediatrician using naloxone, if adequate warning is given.

Case 25

A 42-year-old woman required a hysterectomy for menorrhagia. Over the years her spinal 'arthritis' had resulted in a fixed flexion of the neck and a thoracic kyphosis. She was also being treated for depression with a tricyclic antidepressant.

On examination the patient was observed to be pale. Her neck was fixed in flexion (*Figure 25a*); the tip of the chin was 3 cm from the sternum, and she experienced difficulty looking straight ahead. Full dentition and normal mouth opening were noted. The pulse was 110 beats/min, regular, and the blood pressure was 140/70 mmHg. First and second heart sounds were heard plus an early diastolic murmur best heard over the fourth right intercostal space. The chest showed poor expansion bilaterally, and fine crepitations were audible over both lung bases. Laboratory find-

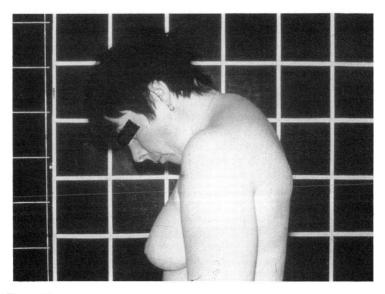

Figure 25a

ings were haemoglobin 5.2 g/dl, mean corpuscular volume 65 fl, mean corpuscular haemoglobin 15 pg, white cell count $7.2 \times 10^9/l$, platelets $344 \times 10^9/l$. The chest X-ray is shown in *Figure 25b* and spirometry results in *Table 25a*.

Questions

1. Describe the anaemia and suggest a cause.
2. What is the rheumatological diagnosis? What other features support the diagnosis?
3. Why is there likely to be a defect in the spirometry?
4. Do you think a regional technique is a practical proposition for this patient's hysterectomy?
5. What must be considered in the treatment of any resulting hypotension?
6. What is the major problem associated with general anaesthesia? Outline in principle how you would deal with this, and indicate the major hazards.

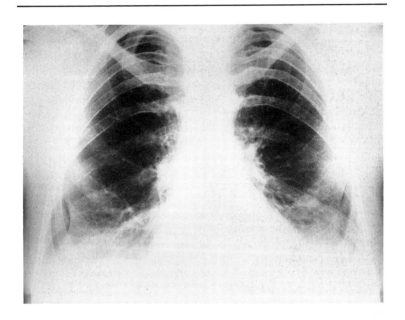

Figure 25b

Table 25a   Results of spirometric testing

	Measured	Predicted
FEV$_1$	1.5	2.2
Vital capacity (litres)	1.8	2.9

Discussion

This woman has a severe hypochromic and microcytic anaemia, undoubtedly due to iron deficiency as a result of her menorrhagia.

The rheumatological diagnosis is ankylosing spondylitis, which chiefly involves the axial skeleton and ultimately leads to a severe flexion deformity and bony ankylosis of the entire vertebral column. It is comparatively rare in women, 90% of affected individuals being male. However, this woman illustrates the multi-system nature of the disease in that she shows pulmonary fibrosis, although this is classically said to involve the upper lobes, and has the murmur of aortic regurgitation due to the associated aortitis.

Clearly this patient could not be intubated in the conventional fashion, and on first consideration regional anaesthesia (either spinal or epidural) might be regarded as the method of choice. However, bony ankylosis of the vertebral column may make this technically impossible, and even if correctly placed, reliable and predictable spread of the local anaesthetic solution would be difficult to guarantee within the deformed spinal canal. A further consideration is the concurrent administration of the tricyclic antidepressant. This means that the use of indirectly acting sympathomimetics such as ephedrine, whose action depends upon uptake into the adrenergic nerve terminal, would be ineffective in the treatment of hypotension. It would be necessary to employ a direct-acting α-adrenergic agonist such as methoxamine.

The disease process leads to bony ankylosis of the costochondral junctions, a rigid chest wall and a reduction in the vital capacity. The fusion of the costotransverse joints is difficult to see on the chest radiograph, but the increase in the basal lung markings is compatible with fibrotic lung disease. This is supported by the spirometry which illustrates a restrictive defect (*Table 25a*).

General anaesthesia poses a number of problems, but above all others is the difficulty in securing the airway with an endotracheal tube. As one could not reliably guarantee either to maintain the airway with the patient breathing spontaneously or to ventilate by hand using a bag and mask, the method of choice would be some form of awake intubation by means of a fibreoptic bronchoscope. This could be achieved nasally or via the oral route using a split pharyngeal airway.

Consideration should be given to antisialogogue premedication and the judicious use of sedative agents during the procedure to improve patient tolerance, but not so excessive as to impair cooperation. Pulse oximetry is particularly valuable when performing fibreoptic intubations. Local anaesthesia of the oropharynx is generally achieved with 4% lignocaine spray, remembering that rapid systemic absorption from this site will predispose to toxicity if excessive doses are used. Patient, careful spraying under direct vision may obviate the need for special techniques to block the external branch of the superior laryngeal nerve in the piriform fossa, or cricothyroid injection to block the internal (sensory) branch of the recurrent laryngeal nerve. If it is thought necessary to block the internal branch of the superior laryngeal nerve this is done by locating the lower border of the hyoid bone laterally and 'walking' off this with a needle; ideally there should be a slight loss of resistance on passing through the thyrohyoid membrane. After careful aspiration (you are in the proximity of the carotid sheath), 2 ml of local anaesthetic solution is injected. Another interesting possibility is the administration of nebulized lignocaine prior to the procedure.

At the end of the procedure rapid recovery of consciousness is desirable. The precise technique for maintaining anaesthesia is probably not critical, but a good quality of recovery might be achieved using a step-down infusion of propofol (10 mg/kg/h for 10 minutes, 8 mg/kg/h for 10 minutes and 6 mg/kg/h thereafter). This is a guide to the infusion rate, which is in practice titrated against the response to surgical stimulation in the same way as one would do with a volatile agent, to avoid awareness.

This patient's aortic regurgitation will be made more pronounced by the compensatory increase in cardiac output due to her chronic anaemia. Transfusion should take place several days preoperatively, aiming for a haemoglobin concentration of at least 10–11 g/dl to improve her oxygen flux.

General considerations such as care with positioning, avoidance of nerve palsies and stresses on joints should be particularly emphasized in patients of this type.

Case 26

An 18-year-old man had been a known asthmatic since the age of 3 years. He was an atopic individual with frequent episodes of intermittent wheeze but had never previously required hospital admission. His regular medication consisted of inhaled salbutamol as required and aminophylline (Phyllocontin) 225 mg twice daily. He was admitted to the accident and emergency department having become progressively breathless and unable to speak over the preceding 4 hours.

On examination the patient was found to have a regular pulse of 130 beats/min and blood pressure of 160/100 mmHg with 40 mmHg of paradox; heart sounds were normal. Respiratory features noted were tachypnoea (50 breaths/min), mild cyanosis, accessory muscles of ventilation in use, tracheal tug and rib recession;

percussion note equal and bilaterally resonant; poor air entry bilaterally, with faint expiratory wheeze also audible bilaterally. The tongue was furred and dry. Peak expiratory flow rate (poor cooperation) was around 60 l/min.

Questions

1. What two investigations are vital to the assessment, and why?
2. What would your immediate treatment be, and why? What limitations does the patient's concurrent therapy place on you?
3. Would the following arterial blood gas values on 24% oxygen alter your management?

    pH 7.30, Po_2 8.2 kPa, Pco_2 6.7 kPa, base excess -5 mmol/l

4. Under what circumstances would you elect to ventilate this patient? What would be the characteristics of the ideal ventilator, and what would you aim to achieve with the settings?
5. After a 24-hour period of mechanical ventilation the patient still has tight bronchospasm despite full treatment with intravenous steroids, nebulized and intravenous salbutamol and ipratropium bromide. Arterial blood gas values are as follows:

    pH 7.05, Pco_2 11.8 kPa, Po_2 14.9 kPa, base excess -7 mmol/l

    What other therapeutic options could be considered at this stage?

Discussion

Contrary to what might be anticipated, the mortality from asthma in young patients has risen in recent years, probably representing an increased prevalence of the condition. The majority of young asthmatics are atopic, i.e. they have an autosomal dominant predisposition to generate IgE antibodies to common allergens. Bronchial constriction is initiated when an allergen binds to surface IgE on the bronchial mast cell leading to degranulation of the mast cell and mediator release. These vasoreactive and bronchoreactive mediators are responsible for the early phase of airway obstruction. However, the aetiology of the later stage of airway obstruction is largely inflammatory and it is possible to demonstrate increased numbers of mast cells and eosinophils infiltrating the bronchial wall. In more chronic asthmatics with an element of fixed airways obstruction, subepithelial fibrosis can be demonstrated as the result of proliferating myofibroblasts. Inhaled corticosteroids are probably underused in the maintenance treatment of asthma.

For the most part the assessment of the severity of an acute asthma attack is clinical. However, a chest X-ray should be performed to exclude a pneumothorax, whilst arterial blood gases will indicate the degree of hypoxaemia and whether the patient is beginning to tire and retain carbon dioxide.

Initial treatment should consist of the administration of oxygen in high concentrations. Unlike the elderly patient with chronic bronchitis, these patients are not dependent on hypoxia for their respiratory drive and hypercapnia will generally be the result of respiratory muscle fatigue rather than a failure of central chemoreceptor drive.

First-line treatment is nebulized salbutamol (5 mg in normal saline). This should be delivered via a high concentration of oxygen as the β-adrenergic dilator effects on the pulmonary vasculature may well precede and exceed the bronchodilator effect, worsening the shunt and causing an initial deterioration in Po_2. The salbutamol should be combined with nebulized ipratropium bromide (0.5 mg in normal saline), an anticholinergic agent which will block any parasympathetic tone within the bronchi. It has been traditional to give loading doses of aminophylline (5 mg/kg) in this situation, but there is now increasing awareness of the toxicity of aminophylline to both the cardiovascular and central nervous systems, and this is particularly relevant in this case where the patient has been receiving oral theophyllines. The wisest approach would be continuous nebulized salbutamol, and if there is no response, switching to salbutamol intravenously. If aminophylline boluses and infusions are used they should be governed by frequent blood levels (aiming for 10–20 mg/l) in view of the narrow therapeutic ratio. Hydrocortisone should be administered, and dehydration corrected as this will facilitate the clearance of inspissated secretions.

The hypercapnia per se does not indicate the need for immediate ventilation, but a rising Pco_2 does indicate that the patient is tiring. First-line treatment should be given, blood gases retaken and the patient reassessed. Failure of response, increasing tiredness, the ominous 'silent chest' and persisting or worsening hypercapnia would indicate the need for a period of artificial ventilation.

Most anaesthetists would perform a rapid sequence induction applying cricoid pressure and using suxamethonium preceded by an induction agent — possibly etomidate in view of its cardiovascular stability and minimal propensity to release histamine. Deep halothane anaesthesia in 100% oxygen with topical lignocaine to the vocal cords has been advocated. However, this is technically harder to achieve, particularly in a very anxious and agitated patient. Furthermore, the diminished alveolar ventilation will make it slower and more difficult to achieve an adequate depth of anaesthesia. Sedation could typically be achieved with midazolam by infusion (avoiding morphine due to its histamine releasing effect). Paralysis may be required to facilitate ventilation; vecuronium being the drug of choice. Remember that paralysis will mask any fitting that may result from aminophylline toxicity, making theophylline levels particularly important if paralysis is induced.

These patients may be very difficult to ventilate effectively. The ideal ventilator should be volume preset, time cycled and pressure limited with the facility to vary the I:E ratio, e.g. the Servo 900C. The primary aim is to oxygenate the patient adequately, whilst endeavouring to keep the peak inflation pressures as low as possible and minimize the risk of barotrauma (typically aim to keep below 60 cmH$_2$0). It is not necessary to achieve normocapnia; indeed attempts to achieve this by increasing the peak inflation pressures in an attempt to deliver a greater minute volume may be entirely counterproductive as the high intrathoracic pressures will simply compress pulmonary blood vessels resulting in an increase in the physiological dead space and worsening CO_2 clearance. It is important to allow the alveoli time to empty in expiration. This may be achieved by using relatively slow rates of ventilation and modification of the I:E ratio and tidal volume. Very little of the peak inflation pressure is in fact transmitted to the alveoli, but it is always possible that high pressures could be transmitted via pathways of low resistance such as bullae and a high index of suspicion for pneumothorax should be maintained whenever these patients are ventilated. If the time allowed for expiration is too short this may give rise to the phenomenon of 'auto-PEEP', and it is important not to allow the chest to become progressively hyperexpanded; a simple tape measure by the bedside is a useful expedient.

The 24-hour blood gas values indicate a failure to relieve the bronchospasm. The persisting acidosis may render the patient unresponsive to catecholamines such as intravenous salbutamol and the role of bicarbonate administration in this situation is controversial. Although bicarbonate will increase carbon dioxide production, proponents would argue that this is more than offset by the increased efficacy of treatment and relief of spasm. Both halothane and ketamine are bronchodilators and may have a role therapeutically as well as being alternative forms of sedation. There are reports showing ketamine to be of value, but its emergence side-effects should be borne in mind as should the fact that in the presence of maximal sympathetic stimulation the direct effect of ketamine on the myocardium is depressant. Halothane in the presence of hypercarbia and acidosis is a potent arrhythmogenic agent (consider also methods of administration, scavenging and ideally monitoring of the inspired concentration). High-dose IV salbutamol and bicarbonate therapy are likely to result in the rapid development of hypokalaemia and there is a need for frequent serum potassium estimations.

Bronchoalveolar lavage is another controversial possibility but it can lead to hypoxia both during and after its performance. Acetylcysteine may be delivered directly to mucus plugs to induce their lysis.

Case 27

Listed below are six very typical patients presenting for elective surgical procedures. Assume the following standard investigations are available to you: haemoglobin, urea and electrolytes, ECG and a chest X-ray. Decide which of these investigations you would ideally require to be available prior to surgery and anaesthesia.

Patient 1 is a fit woman of 40 who has menorrhagia due to a fibroid uterus and is to undergo an elective abdominal hysterectomy. She is on no medication and physical examination is unremarkable.

Patient 2 is a fit 65-year-old man presenting for a right inguinal hernia repair. Physical examination is again unremarkable and he is on no medication.

Patient 3 is a 72-year-old chronic bronchitic. He is breathless after walking some 100 metres on the flat, but having stopped smoking in the last 2 years (although not having improved) he has become no worse. He is admitted as a day case for his 6-monthly check cystoscopy. An ECG and chest X-ray are available from his previous admission.

Patient 4 is an entirely healthy 7-year-old boy who requires an orchidopexy.

Patient 5 is a fit 35-year-old woman with a lump in the breast requiring an excision biopsy. On examination the house officer notes, and you confirm, reduced air entry at the right base.

Patient 6 is a woman 55 years old who has hypertension treated with a thiazide diuretic resulting in good control (150/90 mmHg). She has an otherwise uneventful past medical history but now requires a total hip replacement.

Discussion

The author's own suggestions as to where investigation would be appropriate are shown in *Table 27a*, although there will be a wide divergence of opinion amongst anaesthetists. There is no doubt that a vast number of patients are needlessly overinvestigated. As a general principle investigations should only be used where they are likely to reveal information of significance to the conduct of the anaesthesia or the postoperative management that cannot reliably be obtained by clinical history and examination.

In the first patient, who requires a hysterectomy, anaemia may well be present due to chronic blood loss. She may require

Table 27a

Patient	Hb	U&E	ECG	CXR
1	+	−	−	−
2	−	−	−	−
3	−	−	−	−
4	−	−	−	−
5	+	−	−	+
6	+	+	?	−

preoperative transfusion if haemoglobin levels are very low; if they are not low enough to necessitate postponement or preoperative transfusion, they will serve as a guide to intraoperative and postoperative blood requirements.

The second patient, although 65 years old, is healthy and has no cause either to be anaemic or to have an electrolyte abnormality. It is often argued that 'baseline' ECGs should be performed on patients of this age even in the absence of any symptoms or signs suggestive of ischaemic heart disease. However, ECGs are very insensitive detectors of myocardial ischaemia and, indeed, critical occlusive coronary artery disease may be present with an entirely normal ECG. Ask yourself the question: would the presence of asymptomatic ST segment depression alter the conduct of your anaesthetic. There is certainly no reason to perform a chest X-ray.

The third patient has severe chronic obstructive airways disease; however, you are aware of this clinically and have the benefit of previous investigations including a chest X-ray. As his condition has remained stable there is little point in repeating his CXR as it will not tell you anything that you do not already know.

A healthy 7-year-old child clearly has no indication for an ECG or a chest X-ray. Similarly 'routine bloods' will supply no useful information and are merely distressing for the child.

The fifth patient, who has a lump in the breast, has signs in the chest and therefore warrants a chest X-ray for their elucidation. The fear is that she has disseminated carcinoma of the breast resulting in a malignant pleural effusion. With the possibility of disseminated disease a haemoglobin assessment would be useful to exclude anaemia.

Patient 6 is being treated for hypertension with a thiazide diuretic. These drugs may cause hypokalaemia if administered without potassium supplementation, and it would be prudent to have an estimation of the urea and electrolyte levels prior to embarking upon anaesthesia. A reasonable case can be made for a preoperative ECG in this patient to see if the hypertension has resulted in left ventricular hypertrophy. Once again I feel there is no indication to perform a chest X-ray; but others may well differ.

Overinvestigation of patients has the greatest propensity for morbidity and certainly cost when chest X-rays are considered. The Royal College of Radiologists' guidelines (*Table 27b*) indicate that these films are only useful when certain specific clinical indications are met, and it is now generally agreed that 'baseline' chest X-rays are a valueless concept.

Table 27b **Guidelines for preoperative chest X-ray use among patients admitted for elective non-cardiopulmonary surgery**

'Routine' preoperative chest X-ray is no longer justified. However, preoperative chest radiography may be clinically desirable in certain patients in the following categories:

(i)   those with acute respiratory symptoms
(ii) those with possible metastases
(iii) those with suspected or established cardiorespiratory disease who have not had a chest radiograph in the previous 12 months
(iv) recent immigrants from countries where tuberculosis is still endemic who have not had a chest radiograph within the previous 12 months

Case 28

A school teacher 1.49 m (4 ft 9 in) tall was advised by her obstetrician to have an elective Caesarean section for the delivery of her first baby, who was lying in the breech position. She was otherwise healthy and the pregnancy had been totally normal save for the problems of an 'unfavourable pelvis'. She wanted a full discussion of the options open to her in terms of the anaesthetic and to be able to make her decision fully aware of the advantages and disadvantages of being 'awake' or 'asleep'.

Questions

1. How would you guide her towards her decision?
2. If she were to choose regional anaesthesia, would you favour spinal (subarachnoid) anaesthesia or an epidural technique? What are the advantages and disadvantages of each?

Discussion

This woman is to undergo an elective caesarean section, and in the absence of any strong obstetric considerations favouring regional or general anaesthesia it is reasonable to allow the patient a considerable degree of choice in the anaesthetic technique, once she has been appraised of the advantages and disadvantages of each.

Basic history taking and clinical examination should reveal if there are any particularly pressing reasons for favouring either method. Obvious disease states such as malignant hyperpyrexia trait or suxamethonium sensitivity would favour avoidance of general anaesthesia. Similarly a bleeding tendency or local sepsis would contraindicate a regional block.

The woman should be reassured that either method has a very high record of safety in experienced hands, but having said that, there is little doubt that regional techniques have an unrivalled safety record; indeed, in the most recent confidential enquiry into maternal deaths, none was attributable to regional techniques performed for Caesarean section. However, there may well be some element of artefact in so far that regional techniques tend to be performed in the better centres where there exists an enthusiasm and commitment toward obstetric anaesthesia. The same may not always be the case when emergency Caesarean sections are performed under general anaesthesia in other circumstances. The majority of the deaths attributable to general anaesthesia occur in the setting of a difficult or failed intubation of the trachea resulting in oesophageal intubation and/or the pulmonary aspiration of acidic gastric contents.

There is no doubt by practitioners of regional anaesthesia for Caesarean section that the resulting neonate is delivered in a better condition following a regional block. This is not an effect of asphyxia on the fetus during general anaesthesia, as umbilical artery pH values have been shown to be similar in both groups, and so the difference must be attributable to the depressant effects of anaesthetic agents on the newborn.

An additional consideration is the reduced incidence of thromboembolic problems associated with regional anaesthesia.

The obvious advantages, then, of a regional technique are that the rare but potentially life-threatening risks to the mother are avoided and that the relatively transitory effects of neonatal depression are prevented. Additionally, the regional technique permits the psychological advantages to the mother of being able to participate in the birth of her baby.

The mother should, however, be aware of the complications of a regional technique and have the procedure fully explained beforehand so she knows what to expect. She should be aware of the requirement for a drip to combat falls in blood pressure, but that these are very readily dealt with if they do occur. The most important side-effect to mention is the possibility of mild to moderate headache following a subarachnoid block or severe headache following an epidural block in the event of a dural tap. She should be advised that the chance of this latter complication is around 1 in 100. Many patients are fearful of paralysis or other long-term neurological catastrophe associated with the employment of regional blocks, and adequate reassurance should be provided on this front. Similarly, patients with chronic back problems are fearful that these may be exacerbated following an epidural.

It should go without saying that despite the inherent advantages of regional techniques they should not be forced on unwilling mothers who may be fearful or psychologically unprepared for wakefulness during a surgical procedure. It is equally important that no woman should be promised that she will definitely be awake for the birth of her baby; in the best of hands all regional techniques have an incidence of failure, and there is always the possibility of having to convert to a general anaesthetic. Similarly, the patient should be aware that at times during the procedure she will be aware of traction and possibly mild discomfort and nausea, and that it is always possible to institute a general anaesthetic during the course of the procedure. This breakthrough discomfort arises because the entire sensory supply of the operative field is not subserved by sympathetic fibres ascending in the sympathetic splanchnic nerve to the thoracolumbar sympathetic outflow of the spinal cord. A few afferent fibres travel via the vagus, whilst the underside of the diaphragm may be irritated resulting in pain transmitted centrally via the phrenic nerve (C-3,4,5).

If a regional technique is decided upon, then a decision has to be made as to whether this will be a spinal (subarachnoid) or an epidural block. This will often come down to the personal preference of the individual practitioner, but it is possible to define advantages and disadvantages for either method.

In general, spinal anaesthesia is a 'one-shot' technique typically employing heavy bupivacaine. It is quicker to perform and the speed of onset of the block is much more rapid, and is thus definitely preferable when time is of the essence. However, with a single-shot technique there is potential for the block to fail to reach high enough (most practitioners would aim for T-4), or alternatively to ascend too high resulting in profound hypotension and/or diaphragmatic paralysis.

Spinal anaesthesia, however, has the advantage of avoiding any problems associated with local anaesthetic toxicity, whereas the volume and dose of local anaesthetic required to achieve an epidural block to T-4 frequently borders on the limits of toxicity.

Spinal headache is particularly troublesome in obstetric patients and cannot be reliably abolished even by using needles as small as 26 G. Interest has focused on the use of even smaller needles (which inevitably introduces a greater degree of technical difficulty), and also on the use of 'pencil point' needles rather than the conventional cutting edge type.

Extradural techniques where a catheter is inserted into the epidural space are slower to perform but permit the block to be gradually built up to the right level with incremental dosage. Hypotension is arguably easier to deal with as it is slower to develop than when induced by a subarachnoid block. The presence of a catheter allows the opportunity to employ extradural opiates for postoperative pain relief. Continuous spinal blocks with 32-G microcatheters have been described but experience with these is not widespread.

The quality of the block is less predictable with the epidural route where the local anaesthetic solution has to cross the epidural space with its septa and loculations to gain access to the cerebrospinal fluid.

A variety of combined spinal and epidural techniques have been described, but again these increase the complexity of the procedure.

Case 29

A 5-year-old child weighing 15 kg had been anaesthetized for an examination of the postnasal space and the insertion of grommets. She had undergone two previous anaesthetics, one for a previous insertion of grommets and the other for the manipulation of a forearm fracture. She was premedicated with temazepam syrup (5 mg) and was not unduly sedated when brought to the anaesthetic room some 90 minutes later. Anaesthesia had been induced intravenously with thiopentone 125 mg and suxamethonium 20 mg, and a 5.5 mm uncuffed oral endotracheal tube passed. Ventilation was initially supported by hand using an Ayre's T-piece with a fresh gas flow of 6 litres per minute (70% nitrous oxide in oxygen supplemented with 2% isoflurane). The procedure took less than 10 minutes and at the end the anaesthetist noted that the bag was moving spontaneously, extubated the child and transferred her to the recovery area. Five minutes later the recovery staff noted that the child appeared to have an obstructed airway and had become cyanosed. The anaesthetist was recalled and reintubated the patient without recourse to further anaesthetic agents. Following a period of brisk ventilation via the Ayre's T-piece connected to the wall oxygen, the 'colour' of the child returned. The anaesthetist felt that the patient's poor spontaneous effort related to an excess of carbon dioxide having been blown off; and by occasional squeezes of the bag maintained good saturation readings on the pulse oximeter and permitted the build-up of carbon dioxide in order to stimulate respiratory drive. Respiratory effort remained poor, however, and some 90 minutes later the child was still 'pink' but remained deeply unconscious. A second anaesthetist was summoned who connected a peripheral nerve stimulator to the patient, which demonstrated a normal 'train-of-four' response.

Questions

1. What do you think has happened to this child?
2. What immediate investigations or treatments would you perform?

Discussion

At this stage, almost 2 hours after the termination of a short procedure, such profound unconsciousness demands an urgent explanation as it is inconceivable that it is due to an abnormally prolonged effect of sedative anaesthetic agents. The administration of naloxone would be inappropriate as no opiates had been given in the first place; there would seem little point in using flumazenil to antagonize any residual benzodiazepine effect as the child was not heavily sedated prior to induction; and the empirical use of general stimulants such as doxapram, particularly in children, is to be depreciated. The anaesthetist very reasonably checks for the full return of the 'train of four' to establish whether there is still residual neuromuscular blockade as a result of a prolonged action to suxamethonium.

It is not an uncommon trap for the inexperienced to misinterpret the transmission of a vigorous cardiac impulse to the bag of the breathing circuit as poor ventilatory effort. However, 'scoline apnoea' would provide an explanation for prolonged apnoea but not for total unresponsiveness in the presence of a normal train-of-four response. An acute metabolic explanation should be sought and urgent blood gas analysis requested along with a bedside blood test to exclude hypoglycaemia. Another possibility to be borne in mind in the event of the basic investigations being unhelpful is that there has been some intracerebral catastrophe such as an intracranial bleed or the 'unmasking' of an intracerebral tumour, where a spontaneously breathing anaesthetic employing volatile agents has resulted in an acute rise in intracranial pressure in a patient with critical intracerebral compliance. In this event a small increase in the intracerebral volume as a result of hypercapnia and the use of volatile agents could result in increased cerebral blood flow and a resulting large increase in the intracerebral pressure.

Arterial blood gas analysis is performed, giving the following values: Po_2 29 kPa, Pco_2 40 kPa, pH 6.59. What possibilities could explain this sequence of events?

A life-threatening hypercarbia has developed which in itself is more than sufficient to explain deep unconsciousness. The patient must now be adequately ventilated to remove carbon dioxide. As the child is ventilated she begins to move, and arterial gas values some 15 minutes later reveal that the Pco_2 has fallen to 8.6 kPa. Over this period, however, there is a short period of fitting which resolves spontaneously. By 25 minutes she appears sufficiently awake and demonstrates adequate spontaneous respiration to permit removal of the endotracheal tube. Clearly her overnight observation should be in an area that permits frequent careful observation. The next morning she is entirely well. The brief episode of fitting is entirely explicable in terms of the metabolic derangement and/or its rapid correction and does not warrant any further investigation or treatment.

The question remains, however, how did this state of affairs develop? The first possibility to consider is whether the girl could have received carbon dioxide from the anaesthetic machine with the CO_2 rotameter left in the fully 'on' position at 2 litres per minute. Secondly, was the fresh gas flow from the wall oxygen supply used in recovery appropriate for the size of the child when employing a T-piece circuit? Equally important, was the geometry of the circuit correct? The presence of a large dead space between the fresh gas flow and the endotracheal tube would permit the build-up of carbon dioxide due to total rebreathing. Finally, had the patient been adequately ventilated during the period in recovery when the anaesthetist was endeavouring to achieve a build-up of carbon dioxide? Total apnoea will result in an increase in the Pco_2 of around 3 mmHg (0.4 kPa) per minute. Over this period it is quite possible for a patient with healthy lungs and a low basal oxygen consumption to remain perfectly well oxygenated from simple diffusion and the occasional squeezes of the bag; and it is another trap for the unwary to equate good colour and acceptable saturation readings with adequate ventilation.

Suxamethonium sensitivity is, however, not excluded by the presence of a normal train of four 90–120 minutes after administration. In this situation scrutiny of previous anaesthetic records is vital as although the child had received previous anaesthetic agents she may not have received suxamethonium, and her postoperative apnoea remains to be adequately explained.

Plasma is sent to the laboratory and the following results obtained:

Cholinesterase   0.53 IU/litre (26°C) (normal 0.65–1.45 IU/litre)
Dibucaine number   13

How would you interpret these results, and how is suxamethonium sensitivity evaluated in the laboratory?

The evaluation and the interpretation of results from patients found to be sensitive to the effects of suxamethonium is subject to a considerable degree of confusion and misunderstanding. In the normal individual the action of suxamethonium is rapidly terminated by enzymatic cleavage of the molecule under the influence of the enzyme cholinesterase. This enzyme, produced in the liver, has no known physiological function. Its activity, however, may be influenced by a number of factors, notably pregnancy, certain disease states and the concomitant administration of certain drugs, e.g. ecothiopate eye drops and the recently developed bronchodilator bambuterol. (Bambuterol is a good example of a prodrug; it undergoes cleavage by pseudocholinesterase to the active drug terbutaline. During this process the activity of the cholinesterase becomes markedly reduced and any patient taking this drug would be anticipated to exhibit extreme suxamethonium sensitivity.) Production of cholinesterase, as is the case for all proteins, is coded for by the presence of two genes (one maternally and one paternally acquired). The normal or usual gene is signified *E1U* and patients possessing two of these genes would be expected to exhibit a normal response to suxamethonium. Around 4% of the population possess a form of abnormal gene. This may be the so-called abnormal gene ($E1A$) or one of the other recognized variant genes; the silent gene ($E1S$) of the fluoride-resistant gene ($E1F$). More recently newer genotypes j, k and h have come to be recognized.

Not all cases of 'scoline apnoea' will have abnormal genetics. Large epidemiological series suggest that of all cases of prolonged action to suxamethonium investigated, 60% will have an inherited deficiency, 10% will be genetically normal but have reduced activity of the enzyme, and 30% will have normal enzyme activity and normal genetics.

In the case considered here, the activity of the enzyme is reduced and the low value for the dibucaine number indicates the possession of abnormal genetics. Dibucaine is the local anaesthetic cinchocaine, and the test relies on the fact that the normal enzyme is inhibited in its presence. Thus when a 10^{-5} molar solution of dibucaine is added to the serum of a normal patient the activity of the cholinesterase is inhibited by around 80%. This is expressed as a dibucaine number of 80, i.e. a high level of inhibition in a normal patient. However, the activity of the abnormal cholinesterase is not inhibited by dibucaine, and a homozygous patient with a double dose of the abnormal gene i.e. ($E1A/E1A$) will have a low dibucaine number of 10–25. A heterozygote patient ($E1U/E1A$) will exhibit an intermediate degre of inhibition yielding dibucaine numbers typically in the region of 60.

This girl is thus either homozygous for the abnormal gene or possibly possesses the abnormal gene in conjunction with the silent gene $E1S$. About 0.04% of the population are homozygous for the abnormal gene and will demonstrate apnoea following suxamethonium. This is typically of 2–3 hours' duration, but may extend to 15–24 hours. Heterozygotes will show a prolonged apnoeic response of up to 20 minutes.

The fluoride-resistant gene is so called because of the fact that the cholinesterase elaborated by this gene shows differential inhibition when exposed to sodium fluoride rather than dibucaine.

This case illustrates the potential value of putting the question, 'Is there any family history of problems related to anaesthetics?', to the parents of children about to undergo anaesthesia. It is also important to arrange for the testing of other members of the family. In this case the child's sister showed a similar homozygous pattern of extreme sensitivity, with both father and grandfather showing the heterozygous pattern of moderate sensitivity.[*] Proper complete care dictates that the family should receive a full explanation of the nature of this condition; they should be reassured that it is not life-threatening, but the importance of conveying the information to subsequent anaesthetists must be stressed.

Case 30

A 24-year-old primigravida was delivered at 28 weeks' gestation by emergency caesarean section. At the time she had a blood pressure of 180/120 mmHg, headache, hypertension and ankle clonus. She was treated postoperatively with a diazepam infusion (2 mg/h) and hydralazine at 10 mg/h. After 24 hours her level of consciousness deteriorated rapidly over a 4-hour period to the extent that she was barely rousable 4 hours later.

Including her infusions, she had received 3 litres of dextrose saline in the preceding 24 hours.

On examination the patient was found to be grossly oedematous and cyanosed with inspiratory stridor. Her pulse was 130 beats/min, regular; blood pressure was 170/110 mmHg; first and second heart sounds were noted with mid-systolic murmur audible in the aortic area. Cyanosis and stridor were observed, and coarse inspiratory crepitations were heard bilaterally throughout both lung fields. Laboratory investigations gave the following results:

Full blood count: haemoglobin 10.5 g/dl; white cell count 18×10^9/l, platelets 130×10^9/l
Urea and electrolytes: sodium 125 mmol/l, potassium 4.3 mmol/l, chloride 95 mmol/l, bicarbonate 21 mmol/l, urea 9.5 mmol/l
Prothrombin ratio 1.2
Albumin 26 g/dl
Blood gases (air): pH 7.22, Po_2 6.4 kPa, Pco_2 6.7 kPa, HCO_3 21 mmol/l, base deficit -6.2 mmol/l

---

[*] Mother not available for testing but would presumably be heterozygous or homozygous for the gene.

Previous 24-hour urinary protein excretion was 13 g; the urine output was less than 300 ml in the last 12 hours. A central venous pressure line was in situ reading 8 mmHg. A Swan-Ganz catheter was inserted and the following values were obtained:

Pulmonary capillary wedge pressure 18 mmHg
Cardiac output 12.1 l/min (cardiac index 6.05 l/min/m^2)
Systemic vascular resistance 608 dyn.s/cm^5
Oxygen availability 516 ml/min.m^2
Oxygen consumption 90 ml/min.m^2

The chest radiograph is shown in *Figure 30a*.

Questions

1. What is the underlying problem? What other features not exhibited in this patient frequently occur?
2. What are the causes for the blood gas abnormalities?
3. What is the cause of the deteriorating level of consciousness?
4. Would you intubate and ventilate this patient? If so, what precautions would you take?

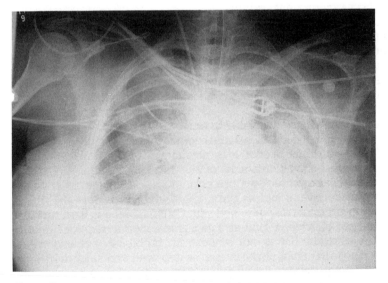

Figure 30a

5. Do you think the Swan-Ganz catheter was necessary? How should this patient be treated?

Discussion

This patient has severe pre-eclampsia. She is hypertensive and grossly oedematous and has now clinically and radiologically developed acute pulmonary oedema. Her deteriorating level of consciousness may in part be due to diazepam therapy or iatrogenic water intoxication, but pre-eclamptic cerebral oedema is the most likely cause. The importance of cerebral oedema is emphasized by the fact that postmortem studies in this group of patients invariably show cerebral oedema associated with microhaemorrhages. The hypoalbuminaemia and the albuminuria are further features of pre-eclamptic toxaemia (PET) and make pulmonary oedema formation more likely at lower levels of left atrial pressure due to the reduction in oncotic Starling forces across the pulmonary capillary bed. However, she does not exhibit the coagulopathy.

Respiratory failure has led to a mixed metabolic and respiratory acidosis. The metabolic component will be due to anaerobic tissue metabolism (possibly due to the marked peripheral oedema) and is suggested by the low value of oxygen consumption despite good oxygen delivery.

The presence of stridor should alert the anaesthetist to the possibility of glottic oedema, whilst the poor gas exchange indicates the need for intubation and ventilation. The positive pressure will encourage the movement of oedema fluid out of the lung, and intubation will protect the airway from the risk of aspiration while the level of consciousness is markedly obtunded. A rapid sequence induction should be performed with a wide range of tube sizes immediately available to combat any glottic oedema.

Although it is well established that central venous pressure (CVP) readings do not give accurate representations of filling pressures on the left side of the heart in severe PET, many relatively uncomplicated pre-eclamptics are treated successfully with vasodilators such as hydralazine, titrating the dose against the blood pressure response and with CVP guidance to fluid replacement or restriction. Hydralazine has assumed a traditional role in this situation but is not without its problems — chiefly reflex tachycardia, tachyphylaxis and nausea with vomiting. Sublingual nifedipine may be a preferable alternative.

It is well recognized that in PET, despite the marked expansion of the extracellular space, there is contraction of the intravascular compartment. Because of this there is likely to be an excessive fall in blood pressure in response to vasodilators unless an adequate circulating volume is maintained; hence the tendency to give a generous preload to pre-eclamptics prior to epidural block. However, this courts the danger of iatrogenic fluid overload, particularly when the CVP is not providing a valuable end point for volume expansion.

Furthermore, post partum there is a large autotransfusion of blood from the uteroplacental bed and mobilization of extracellular fluid into the vascular compartment. In this patient a fair amount of free water has been given which in the face of persisting oliguria will have resulted in a considerable positive fluid balance; a Swan-Ganz catheter is therefore strongly indicated to determine the left-sided filling pressures, whether the circulation is dilated in response to the hydralazine or remains constricted; and furthermore, to indicate whether the cardiac output is high or low. Without this information the choice between fluid, diuretics, inotropes and vasodilators would be little more than guesswork. The position of the Swan-Ganz catheter is not ideal and may not be within a West's zone III position. It should be 'refloated' to lie in the lower zones of the lung fields.

The haemodynamic picture is one of a hyperdynamic, dilated circulation with a high cardiac output and high pulmonary capillary wedge pressure (PCWP). The high PCWP is compatible with the diagnosis of pulmonary oedema. The patient is already vasodilated with a high cardiac output, and further vasodilator therapy to 'offload' the heart would be inappropriate. The urgent need is to remove fluid. A potent loop diuretic such as frusemide should be used in the first instance in the hope that the kidney is able to respond. If it cannot, fluid would have to be removed by dialysis. Fluid should be restricted; concentrated albumin solutions, however, may have a role once diuresis has started by increasing the colloid osmotic pressure of the plasma and facilitating the mobilization of pulmonary, cerebral and peripheral oedema fluid back into the vascular compartment from where it can be removed by the kidney under the influence of diuretics.

Case 31

A 45-year-old woman required a cholecystectomy. She weighed 120 kg and had been diagnosed as a diabetic for 3 years, allegedly treated by diet!

She gave a history of shortness of breath when lying flat and complained of episodic retrosternal chest pain associated with food and bending. She was taking bendrofluazide 10 mg once a day.

Examination revealed a regular pulse of 72 beats/min and blood pressure of 200/120 mmHg. Heart sounds were normal, and the chest was clear. A full blood count gave normal values. Plasma electrolyte levels were: sodium 125 mmol/l, potassium 3.0 mmol/l, chloride 100 mmol/l and bicarbonate 20 mmol/l; urea was 5.0 mmol/l and glucose 22 mmol/l. An ECG (*Figure 31a*) and a chest radiograph (*Figure 31b*) were requested.

Questions

1. What relevant medical problems can be identified?
2. What further investigation, evaluation or treatment would you require prior to surgery and anaesthesia?
3. How would you induce anaesthesia?
4. What type of ventilator would you use?
5. What would be the major concern postoperatively, and how might this be attenuated?

Discussion

Several problems in this case render surgery and anaesthesia particularly hazardous. Firstly there is inadequate control of this patient's diabetes; this should be brought under control preoperatively using regular doses (three times daily) of a short-acting insulin. When the patient is 'nil by mouth', a balanced glucose and insulin infusion should be established with the insulin infusion rate titrated against frequent capillary glucose samples. This regimen should be continued postoperatively until the normal oral intake is re-established. The normal requirements for saline must not be forgotten or else hyponatraemia will develop in the postoperative

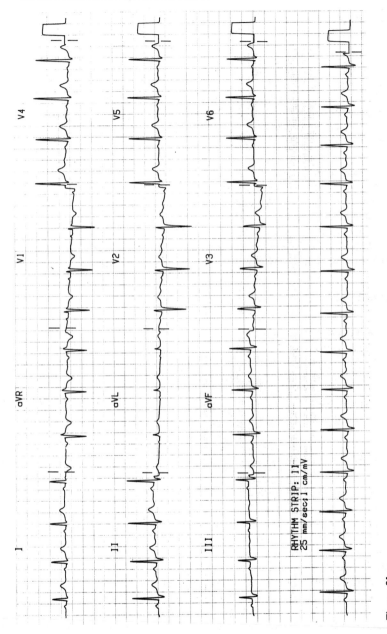

Figure 31a

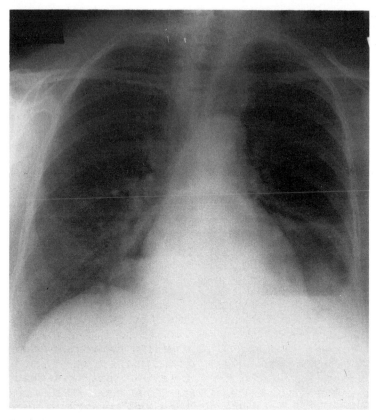

Figure 31b

period. The preoperative hyponatraemia is an appropriate response to the hyperglycaemia and should correct itself as the blood glucose returns to more normal values. The hypokalaemia is probably due to thiazide therapy and the need for this drug should be critically reviewed as it will also tend to exacerbate the diabetic state.

The evaluation of the cardiovascular system is more problematic. The blood pressure reading suggests that this patient is hypertensive; but is she truly hypertensive? Has the blood pressure been taken with an appropriately large cuff? Note that there is no evidence of left ventricular hypertrophy on the ECG to suggest that the left ventricle has been ejecting against an elevated systemic vascular resistance for a prolonged period. A series of readings should be instituted with an appropriately sized cuff and a trend established. If she is hypertensive, treatment should be instituted, and control attained prior to elective surgery. In these circumstances a vasodilator drug such as nifedipine would probably be preferable to a thiazide/beta-blocker combination. Mild orthopnoea in an obese individual does not necessarily equate with heart failure and is most probably related to the increase in the mechanical work of breathing and the reduction in the functional residual capacity. The chest pain does not sound cardiac in origin and there is no evidence of ischaemia on the ECG, but this by no means rules out the possibility of asymptomatic coronary atheroma in an obese diabetic patient. The chest X-ray shows the presence of a hiatus hernia (gas bubble behind the heart shadow) and the history relating to the pain is very suggestive of acid reflux. Preoperative treatment with an H_2-receptor antagonist such as ranitidine will raise the gastric pH and reduce the likelihood of a pulmonary acid aspiration syndrome developing in the event of regurgitation and aspiration at the induction of anaesthesia.

Because of the incompetence of the lower oesophageal sphincter and the potential difficulty of intubating this patient, a rapid sequence induction using suxamethonium and cricoid pressure would be mandatory. A full range of laryngoscopes including a 'polio' blade should be to hand, along with other aids to intubation such as gum elastic bougies. A highly lipid-soluble agent such as thiopentone, which relies largely on redistribution for its termination of action, will be very widely redistributed in the obese individual and there may be a prolonged hangover period. A more rapidly metabolized induction agent such as propofol or etomidate might be preferable.

The reduction in the compliance of the chest may make obese patients impossible to ventilate with popular minute volume divider ventilators such as the Manley. A flow generator type of machine such as the Nuffield Penlon, Servo or Oxford would be more suitable.

The deleterious effects of obesity on respiratory function increase the incidence of episodic hypoxaemia, which may increase the likelihood of a myocardial infarction for several days into the postoperative period. When the obese patient is placed supine the weight of the chest wall and the abdominal contents will have a marked effect on the mechanics of ventilation. Depending on the elasticity of the diaphragm, lung volumes will be reduced, and there will be a greater reduction in the functional residual capacity (FRC) than when the lean individual is transferred from the erect to the supine position. Surgery and anaesthesia will result in a further reduction of the functional residual capacity. Airway closure will occur in normal, young individuals at low lung volumes when intrapleural pressure exceeds the airway pressure. With age there is a progressive loss of the elastic tissue of the lung parenchyma, reducing the ability to hold the airways open; therefore the closing volume tends to rise with age and will encroach upon the resting position. In the obese subject, operating at a lower FRC, this closing volume will more readily encroach upon (and exceed) the FRC and lead to an increased alveolar–arterial oxygen difference during tidal breathing. At low lung volume the patient is at an unfavourable (non-compliant) point on the pressure–volume curve of the lung and the work of breathing will be increased. Postoperative pain will compound the problem by inhibiting the ability to breathe deeply, resulting in the development of basal atelectasis. Oxygen therapy should be continued for several days into the postoperative period, and ideally the haemoglobin saturation should be monitored by means of a pulse oximeter.

The problem may be attenuated, but not entirely abolished, by a more imaginative approach to postoperative analgesia. A thoracic epidural blockade would probably be the ideal solution, but may be technically difficult to perform in the obese individual. Other possibilities are intercostal nerve blocks or possibly the insertion of an intrapleural catheter and the infusion of a local analgesic solution.

Regular physiotherapy should not be forgotten.

Index

Abdominal pain, 42
  in sickle cell anaemia, 42, 43
Acid aspiration syndrome, 28,
  29, 93, 121
Acromegaly, 86, 87, 89, 90
Acute laryngotracheal
  bronchitis, 17
Adrenocorticotrophic hormone
  (ACTH), 90
Adult respiratory distress
  syndrome, 36
Allergy, 80
Anaemia, 1, 42
  from fibroid, 104
  iron deficiency, 97
  of renal failure, 2
Anaesthesia:
  for day care surgery, 20
  family history and, 113
  hypersensitivity to, 80, 81
  for malignant hyperpyrexia
    syndrome, 62, 63
  one lung, 58
  See also under conditions,
    lesions etc.
Anaesthetics:
  hypersensitivity to, 80, 81
Analgesia:
  in labour, 24, 26
  postoperative, 11, 122
Anaphylaxis, 80, 81
Angina, 6
Anion gap, 52
Ankle blocks, 5
Ankylosing spondylitis, 96, 97
Antibodies for septicaemia, 38
Anticoagulant therapy, 77

Antidiuretic hormone, 91
Aorta:
  dissection of, 58
  double-barrelled, 58
  tears in, 22
Aortic aneurysm:
  abdominal, 6
  prognosis, 9
Aortic regurgitation, 95, 99
Arthroscopy, 39
Ascites, 46
Aspiration pneumonitis, 78, 79,
  see also Acid aspiration
  syndrome
Aspirin, 92
Asthma, 99
  acute attack, 101
Atlantoaxial subluxation, 3

Blood transfusion in sickle cell
  disease, 44
Bowel resection, 45
Brain:
  ischaemia, 51
  oedema, 74, 116
Breast:
  biopsy of, 104, 105
Bronchitis, 103
Bronchoalveolar lavage, 103
Bronchospasm, 79, 80, 100, 102
Bronchus:
  rupture of, 31

Caesarean section, 106, 114
  anaesthesia for, 93, 94, 106,
  107
Captopril, 7

Carbon dioxide accumulation, 61, 111, 112
Cardiac tamponade, 32
Carpal tunnel syndrome in pregnancy, 26, 37
Central nervous system:
  ethylene glycol intoxication of, 54
Cerebral accidents:
  in pregnancy toxaemia, 95
Cerebral ischaemia, 51
Cerebral oedema, 74
  pre-eclamptic, 116
Chest:
  injuries to, 30, 66
Chest pain, 55, 118
  in hiatus hernia, 121
  postoperative, 20, 22
Chest X-rays:
  indications for, 104, 105, 106
Cholecystectomy, 118
Circulatory collapse in babies, 63, 65
Cirrhosis, 46
Coagulopathy, 47
Colloid oncotic pressure, 68
Colloids, 66, 68
Coronary artery bypass, 10
Crohn's disease, 45
Croup, 17
Cuff herniation, 79
Cyanosis, 60
  during anaesthesia, 110
  in crush injury, 30
  traumatic, 66

Dantrolene, 62
Day care surgery, 19, 21
Deafness, postoperative, 20, 21
Deep vein thrombosis, 48, 51
Dehydration, 42
  in babies, 63, 64
Dental surgery, 19, 21

Desmopressin, 91
Diabetes insipidus, 91
Diabetes mellitus, 118
Disseminated intravascular coagulation, 35
Diverticulum, perforated, 32
Dyspnoea, 118
  in airways disease, 82
  in asthma, 99
  in mitral stenosis, 74, 76
  in pregnancy, 22

Ectopic beats, 70, 71
Electrocardiography:
  indications for, 104, 105
Electrolytes;
  during pregnancy, 28
  in pyloric stenosis, 64
Emphysema, 88
Encephalopathy:
  hepatic, 74
Endobronchial intubation, 79
Epiglottitis;
  acute, 17
Epilepsy, 19
  anaesthesia and, 21
Ethylene glycol intoxication, 54
Extradural techniques, 109
Eye:
  pain in, 48

Faecal peritonitis, 32
Fat embolism, 69
Felty's syndrome, 3
Femur:
  fracture of, 66
Fetus:
  anaesthesia and, 94
Flail chest, 30, 66
Flumazenil, 73
Flunitrazepam:
  overdose of, 70

Fractures:
early fixation of, 69

Gallstones, 42
Gastric reflux, 29, 80, 121
Gelofusine, 68
Glasgow coma scale, 71, 72
Glottic oedema, 116
Goldman cardiac risk index, 9

Haemacel, 67, 68, 69
Haemodiafiltration, 14
Haemofiltration, 14
Haemolytic anaemia, 43
Halothane:
hyperpyrexia and, 62
Heart murmurs:
in mitral stenosis, 77
in pregnancy, 27
Heart strain, 39, 55, 58
Hepatitis B, 47
Hepatorenal syndrome, 47
Hernia repair, 103
Hetastarch, 67, 68
Hiatus hernia, 29, 80, 121
Hip replacement, 74, 78, 104
Hyperbilirubinaemia, 44
Hypercarbia, 61, 111, 112
Hyperglycaemia, 120
Hypersensitivity to
anaesthesia, 80, 81
Hypertension, 6, 55, 104, 105,
120
in pre-eclamptic toxaemia,
114
pulmonary, 24, 39, 43, 78
Hyperventilation, 51
Hypoglycaemia, 42
Hypotension, 35
induced, 49, 50
Hypoxia, 66
Hysterectomy, 95, 103, 104
anaesthesia for, 96, 98

Imipramine:
overdose, 70
Inotropes, 35, 38
Intracranial aneurysms, 50
surgery for, 50
Intubation:
in children, 18
endobronchial, 79
hypertensive response
during, 95
Ion trapping phenomenon, 28
Ischaemic heart disease, 105
anaesthesia and, 11
oxygen therapy and, 12

Jaundice, 43

Kidney:
effect of drugs on, 2, 3, 6
protection of, 47, 48
Kyphosis, 95
anaesthesia in, 98

Labour, anaesthesia in, 26
Laryngeal nerve palsy, 22, 24,
25
Laryngotracheal bronchitis, 17
Left bundle branch block, 88,
90
Left ventricular hypertrophy,
55
Liver:
failure, 46
paracetamol necrosis, 73, 74
Lung;
fibrotic disease of, 98

Malignant hyperpyrexia
syndrome, 61, 107
Metabolic acidosis, 52
Mitral stenosis, 75, 76
spinal anaesthesia in, 77
Muscle physiology, 61

Myalgia, suxamethonium, 22
Myocardial infarction, 6, 13, 121
  postoperative, 13

Neonate:
  respiratory depression in, 95
Nitrous oxide:
  teratogenic effect of, 29
Non-steroidal
    anti-inflammatory drugs:
  mode of action, 5
  side effects of, 1
Nuclear magnetic resonance, 86, 89, 90

Obesity:
  respiratory function and, 121
Obstructive airways disease, 84, 105
Oesophageal sphincter:
  anaesthesia and, 121
Oesophagus:
  intubation of, 60
Oliguria:
  postoperative, 12
One lung anaesthesia, 58
Opiates:
  side effects of, 13
Orchidopexy, 104
Osmolar gap, 52
Osteoarthritis, 74
Oxygen consumption, 37, 38
Oxygen therapy, 12, 122

Palpitation, 52, 53, 55
Paracetamol:
  metabolism, 72
  overdose, 70
Paroxysmal nocturnal
    haemoglobinuria, 51
Pink puffers, 84
Pituitary adenoma, 89

Pituitary hormones, 90
Pneumonia, recurrent, 42
Pneumothorax, 79, 82, 101
  in acromegaly, 90
  traumatic, 30, 67
Porphyria, 41, 42
Portal hypertension, 46
Posterior communicating artery:
  aneurysm of, 49
Postnasal space:
  examination of, 109
Pre-dilution, 15
Pre-eclamptic toxaemia, 92, 114
Pregnancy:
  anaesthesia in, 26, 91, 93
  carpal tunnel syndrome in, 26
  dyspnoea in, 22
  electrolytes in, 28
  heart murmurs in, 27
  'normal' measurement in, 27
  pulmonary hypertension in, 26
  toxaemia of, 91, 92, 114
Prostacyclin, 15
Pulmonary hypertension, 24, 39, 78
  in sickle cell disease, 43
Pulmonary oedema, 13, 117
  in toxaemia of pregnancy, 94, 116
  low pressure, 36
  paracetamol causing, 74
Pyloric stenosis, 64

Rectum:
  carcinoma of, 81
Renal disease:
  arterial surgery and, 13
Renal failure, 2
  paracetamol causing, 74
  postoperative, 12, 14

in toxaemia of pregnancy,
92
Respiratory failure:
in pre-eclamptic toxaemia,
116
Respiratory tract infection, 16
Rheumatic fever, 74, 76
Rheumatoid arthritis, 1
Right bundle branch block, 39,
70, 71
Road traffic accident, 66
Robertshaw tube, 58

Salbutamol, 101
Scoline apnoea, 110, 113
Septicaemia, 34
treatment of, 38
Shock, 30
septicaemic, 34, 38
Sickle-cell disease, 43
surgery in, 44
Spinal anaesthesia:
in Caesarean section, 108
in mitral stenosis, 77
rheumatoid arthritis and, 5
Spinal cord:
damage from surgery, 59
transection of, 4
Spinal headache, 109
Splenomegaly, 46, 47
Stavermann reflection
coefficient, 69
Stomach:
effect of NSAIDs on, 2
Stomach content:
aspiration of, 28, 29, 78, 79,
93, 121
Stridor, 114, 116
Subarachnoid haemorrhage, 49

Suxamethonium:
malignant hyperpyrexia
syndrome and, 62
Suxamethonium myalgia, 22
Suxamethonium sensitivity, 107,
112
Systemic vascular resistance,
35

Tachycardia, 60
Teeth extraction, 19
Third nerve palsy, 49
Thoracic aorta:
dissection of, 58
surgery of, 59
Thoracic epidural blockade:
for arterial surgery, 11
Thrombocytopenia, 82
Thumb:
paraesthesia of, 26
Thyroid stimulating hormone,
90
Tracheostomy, 18, 31
Tricyclic antidepressants:
side effects of, 73

Upper airways obstruction, 16
Uterine fibroids, 103

Vasospasm, 50, 51
Ventilation, mechanical, 18, 86
in asthma, 101, 102
Vertabrae:
fracture of, 31
Vision, double, 48

Wenckebach phenomenon, 10
Wolff–Parkinson–White
syndrome, 53, 55